Miriam Stoppard's Healthcare

Miriam Stoppard's

Healthcare

With an A-Z of Common Medical Complaints and How to Treat Them

WEIDENFELD AND NICOLSON
LONDON

Second Impression 1981

Designed by Martin Richards
for George Weidenfeld and Nicolson Limited
91 Clapham High Street, London SW4
Diagrams by Wilcock: Riley Graphic Art Limited

ISBN 0 297 77724 6

Set, printed and bound in Great Britain by
Fakenham Press Limited,
Fakenham, Norfolk

Contents

Introduction

Where do all the healthy, fit and slender twenty-five-year-olds go? Gone to ailing, unfit, paunchy forty-five-year-olds, is too often the unfortunate answer. Why, as a general rule, should health and physical fitness be enjoyed only in the first half of life? Is it inevitable that we thicken and slacken with age? As it patently is not, why do we allow it to happen? Why do we let the rippling muscle turn to fat and the curved waistline straighten and bulge? Despite knowing how important it is to stay fit and healthy we think too rarely about the consequences of becoming unfit. We comfort ourselves with the thought that serious illness happens exclusively to other people. In the absence of illness, health and fitness routines get a very low priority. Above all we are lazy.

Most of us accept that getting older means getting fatter and slower. There are enough examples of people who refuse to equate age with being unfit to make it obvious that none of us needs to. To enter middle age healthy, fit and slim we have to start preparing when we are quite young – under thirty if possible. It is never too late, however, and now is as good a time as any.

The first and most important part of preparation is to find the will and the determination to change your way of life. You really have to care about being healthy and fit; you must have the strength to change many of the ingrained habits in your life and not to weaken. Most of us need a trigger that helps us find the strength and the more dramatic it is the more effective it will be; a severe illness or the death of a friend can make us see our priorities in life quite differently. Once you have found the will there is nothing between you and the joy of having and using a body in peak condition.

The human body is a miraculous machine. The majority of us abuse our bodies and neglect them in a way we would not contemplate with a piece of precious jewellery, even less with a car. Your body deserves attention, care and regular maintenance. To give it less puts your life in jeopardy. So you should be prepared to work very hard to become fit and healthy. If it is statistics you need to prove that health and longevity go hand in hand, there are plenty around. Any insurance actuary will confirm that a healthy person will live longer than an unhealthy one.

If you are healthy you are less prone to disease than when you are unfit and overweight. Conditions involving the joints and the muscles like arthritis, fibrositis, lumbago, low back pain and sciatica, are less common in people who are fit. Chest disease, heart disease, diabetes, eye disease and digestive problems are all found less frequently in people who are fit and healthy than in those who are not, and this applies to almost any disease you can name. The chance of longer life is therefore greater.

More importantly, while you are living that longer, healthier life you will probably be happier. You can get more out of life, you can throw yourself more readily into new activities, you can enjoy yourself more. Your life can become more interesting, more flexible and more adventurous. As a bonus, many of the activities undertaken by fit and healthy people bring them into contact with others, bring them closer to their families, cement relationships and help husbands and wives to join together in mutual interests.

A few months ago I shared the lift of a very expensive, plush, London hotel with a slim, middle-aged gentleman of about fifty-five dressed in a track suit and plimsolls. It was quite a shock to see someone thus dressed in such urbane surroundings. I asked him what he was going to do in the centre of London dressed the way he was. 'I'm going to jog in Hyde Park,' he explained. 'I do it every time I come to London. I check in, change and go straight out into the Park and jog for an hour.' 'You're a confirmed jogger then?' I asked. 'Oh, yes,' he said. 'I've jogged round most of the capitals of the world.'

Our international jogger provides the answer to most of our excuses for not taking exercise – 'I am too busy', 'My life is already overcrowded', 'I have other priorities', 'Many things are more important to me than staying fit'. This determined gentleman, despite his tight schedule of international travel, despite the pressure of business meetings, made time for his jogging. Notwithstanding the stress of his job, I imagine he is happier, calmer and more able to cope with tension and anxiety than his sedentary colleagues. What is more, he is decreasing the chance of succumbing to 'businessman's disease' (a heart attack), unlike the jet-lagged executive who climbs off the aeroplane, takes a taxi to the hotel, settles down to a stiff whisky, has an extended dinner with business friends in the evening, and retires well after midnight.

He also exemplifies the price that you have to pay to remain fit. Staying fit is difficult and uncomfortable, even painful. Staying fit requires great effort, and usually at a time when you least want to make it. The very minimum that is required of you is to eat properly and to exercise regularly and frequently.

There is a difference between *regular* exercise and *frequent* exercise. You have to do both to stay fit. You become healthy by eating properly. You become fit by exercising. To stay fit and healthy you have to eat properly and exercise properly. If you do both you will not, incidentally, have any weight problems.

There is one more commitment to make if you are going to be fit and healthy: you should avoid abusing your body. Alcohol in large quantities is always detrimental to you; smoking, even five cigarettes a day, is harmful to your health and can never be anything else. You are undoubtedly better off without either of them.

All this sounds as if you have to be a fanatic to be fit and healthy. We would all be paragons if we rode a bicycle round the district for fifteen miles before going to work, or jogged for an hour every evening before we went to bed. We would be well nigh perfect if we ate a perfectly balanced diet all the time and did not indulge in the odd bar of chocolate or the large piece of pie with masses of cream. We should not expect, nor should we try, to stick to rigid regimens day in and day out. One of the most important things to face up to is that we all fail now and then and that we will all err sooner or later. Your motto should be that it is better to do some exercise as often as you can rather than not at all. And it is better to control your appetite and eat a well-balanced diet most of the time, accommodating the occasional transgression, than not at all. The other part of the motto is that if you do break the rules, do not throw everything to the wind and abandon your good intentions. One indiscretion does not ruin everything.

An extension of the motto is to do what suits you rather than what people or books tell you you ought to do. While some will swear by rowing machines and dumb-bells, if yoga or transcendental meditation is what you like doing you should go ahead and do it. You are unlikely to stick to something that you do not enjoy. The most important thing is that you take up some form of exercise and adhere to some sort of diet. Choose ones that you feel at home with and you will stand a good chance of being able to carry on with them for the rest of your life.

The pay-off to the motto is that once you have achieved the level of fitness which is right for your age, size and capacity, maintenance of fitness takes very much less effort. While you are getting up to your level of fitness you may have to work very hard and perform your exercises every day for six or eight weeks. Having achieved your level of fitness, however, you will need to go through your exercise schedule no more than three times a week.

Do not be put off by people who say that using an exercise bicycle at home, or doing your stint at the Canadian BX exercises is cheating at getting fit. If an exercise bicycle is what your life can accommodate it is far better than nothing at all. Do whatever your own life and routine allows you to. As long as you stick at it and do not give up, you will achieve your goal of attaining and maintaining health and fitness.

Part and parcel of this theory is that you encourage others around you to keep fit too. Wherever possible you should take up physical activities that involve the family, including your husband or wife. Never discourage your partner from taking exercise, whatever it is. It may not be your idea of fun to try to hit a little ball into a hole for two or three hours every Saturday morning, but it is good for your husband, and you will have him for longer if you encourage him to do it. If you set your children a good example by eating properly and exercising regularly, you will be teaching them good habits for the rest of their lives.

As part of your own fitness campaign try to include some of the following good examples:

1 Get up early in the morning for a jog.

2 Walk or cycle to the shops or work rather than using a car or taking a bus.

3 Walk up the stairs rather than use a lift or an escalator.

4 Make other members of your family feel guilty when you take exercise and they do not.

5 Meet friends for a game of tennis or squash rather than at the pub.

6 Drink alcohol only at mealtimes and always in moderation.

7 Encourage your guests not to take too much alcohol if they are driving home.

8 Do not press food or drinks on other people.

9 Eat lots of fish and vegetables.

10 Do not eat two large meals in a day. If you have a dinner planned for the evening, eat only fruit for lunch, or vice versa.

11 Do not arrange your dinner party menu so that each course has a high fat content.

12 Provide salad and other healthy options as often as you can, particularly for slimmers at dinner parties.

13 Give your family and visitors wholemeal bread with 'soft'-fat margarine rather than white bread and butter.

14 Do not give sweets frequently to your own or other people's children.

15 Do not give chocolates and sweets and cigarettes as presents.

16 Do not smoke without permission if there are other people around.

17 Compliment people on losing weight or on giving up cigarettes.

18 Do not sympathize or agree with people who say they cannot stop smoking or lose weight.

19 Do not compliment a mother on a bonny baby when in fact the baby is fat.

20 Do not regard health as something that only doctors need worry about.

Be healthy – live longer!

How the Body Works

No organ in the body is independent of the rest. It follows that the health of every organ depends on the health of the rest. You can only understand fully how to maintain the health of your body if you understand how the organs work and how they interrelate.

The human body is more beautiful and more efficient than any machine: the brain, for instance, can store more information and work more effectively than a computer; our joints move with less friction than the parts of a man-made engine; we could view the heart, which starts to beat when we are embryos of a few weeks old and continues ceaselessly until we die, as the nearest thing to perpetual motion we are ever likely to see.

In this chapter the organs are grouped into 'systems' because several organs have to work in unison to maintain the efficiency of the body. In practical terms the heart and blood-vessels cannot be separated so they are described together. Sight and hearing are dealt with as integral parts of our sensory system through which we gather information about the external world and adapt ourselves to it. The brain is considered in conjunction with the rest of the nervous system of which it acts as the controller.

No attempt is made to describe the detailed anatomy of different organs but emphasis is given to describing the function of each organ and how that relates to the function of others. In this way I have endeavoured to provide a backcloth for the principles and practices advocated in the rest of the book.

The brain and central nervous system

By far the greatest and heaviest parts of the brain are the cerebral hemispheres, the two large convoluted lobes with an appearance similar to a shelled walnut. They occupy most of the skull, while the rest of the brain takes up very little room. It is the size of the cerebral hemispheres which is responsible for our intelligence and many of the skills which only we human beings enjoy. Only one or two mammals have cerebral hemispheres as large as our own – apes and sea-living mammals such as whales and dolphins – and these animals are probably as intelligent, in absolute terms, as we are.

The word skills – reading, writing and speaking – seeing, hearing, feeling, moving and all intellectual thought processes are contained within the outer-

Outer surface of cerebral hemisphere

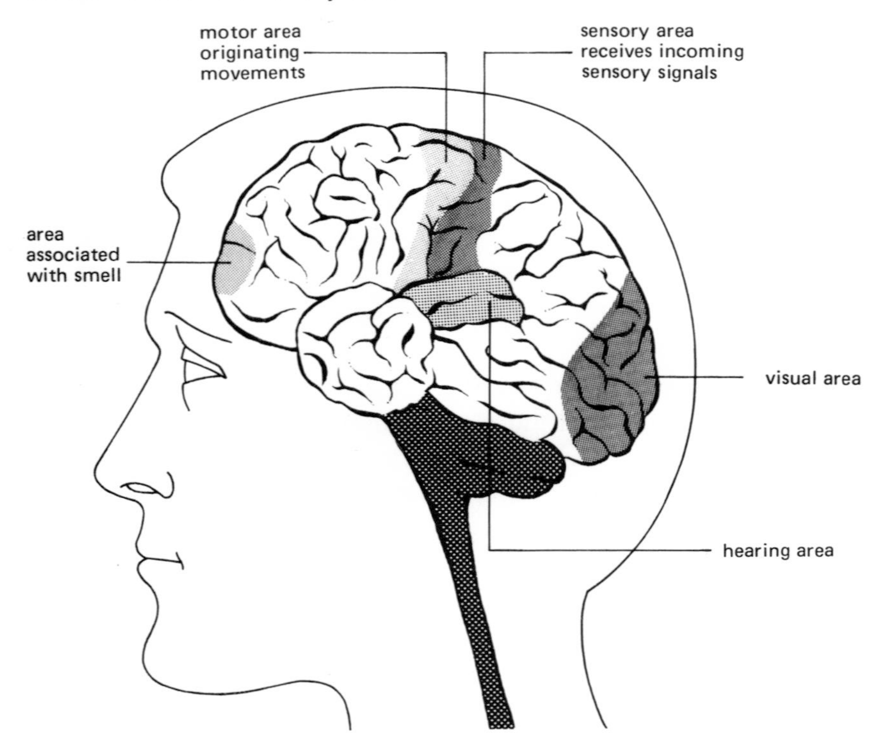

most layer of the cerebral hemispheres – the cerebral cortex, which contains the grey cells.

The other parts of the brain, like the brain stem, the cerebellum and the hypothalamus, though very small in comparison, are concerned with the basic functions that keep us alive.

The brain operates on a massive scale, sending out messages to various parts of the body all the time, in response to a bombardment of messages from various other parts of the body and from the outside world. The messages are chemical or electrical: chemical messages arrive in the blood; electrical messages flash up nerves as electrical charges. An example of a chemical message is a high level of sugar in the blood due to gorging on a huge rich meal. On sensing this the brain sends a message to the pancreas to increase the output of insulin into the blood-stream. The level of insulin increases and the excess sugar is cleared from the blood into the liver and other tissues. The blood sugar returns to normal due to the controlling influence of the brain. An example of an electrical message involving the brain is *seeing* something (see p. 36). An electrical message which by-passes the brain is the sensation of something very hot on your fingers and the immediate withdrawal of your hand from the hot object you are touching.

Before we even feel the pain we reflexively pull back our hands if the fingers are in danger of being burned.

The spinal cord is an extension of the brain and runs down through our spinal bones nearly to the bottom of the back. All the way down the spine, nerves branch off and supply various parts of the body.

Each nerve is split into two parts – a sensory nerve and a motor nerve. The sensory nerves carry messages inwards to the spinal column, and on to the brain if appropriate. These messages are in the form of sensations picked up by the skin in the form of heat, cold, touch and pain, and also from the joints in the form of information about limb movements. The motor nerves carry messages outwards and they activate the muscles. An electrical impulse passing down a motor nerve would, by the release of a chemical, cholinesterase, cause a muscle to contract and therefore move a limb or joint.

The brain controls a secondary nervous system, called the autonomic nervous system, which is connected to the internal organs, and affects the emptying

Slice through the brain

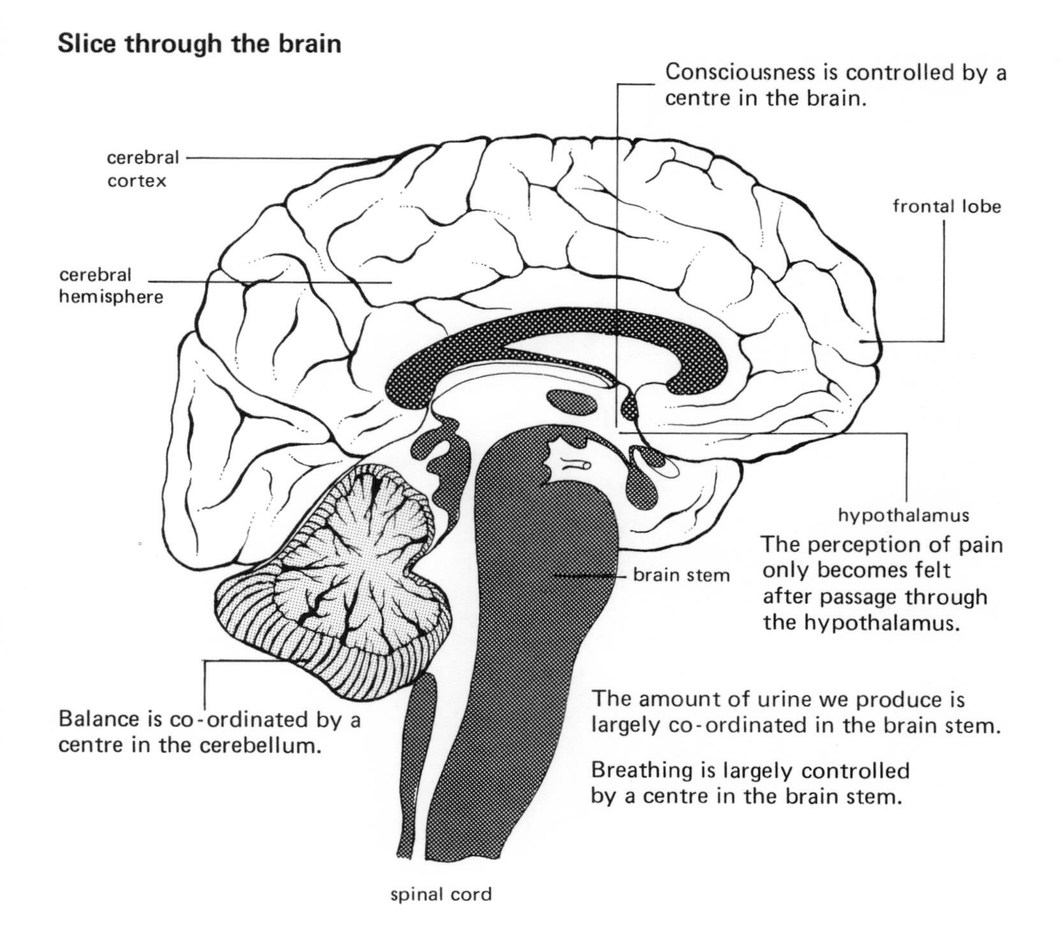

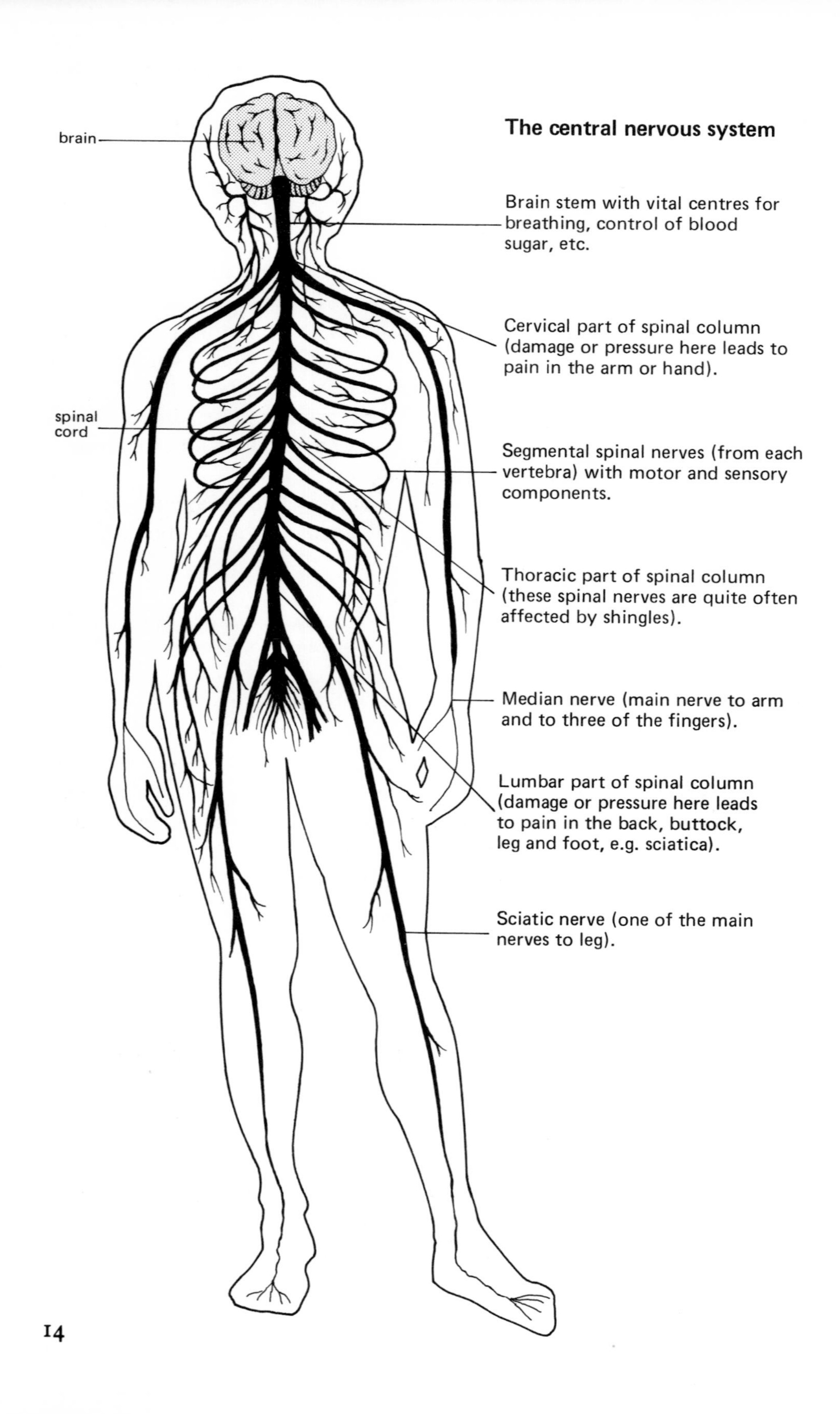
brain
spinal cord
The central nervous system
Brain stem with vital centres for breathing, control of blood sugar, etc.
Cervical part of spinal column (damage or pressure here leads to pain in the arm or hand).
Segmental spinal nerves (from each vertebra) with motor and sensory components.
Thoracic part of spinal column (these spinal nerves are quite often affected by shingles).
Median nerve (main nerve to arm and to three of the fingers).
Lumbar part of spinal column (damage or pressure here leads to pain in the back, buttock, leg and foot, e.g. sciatica).
Sciatic nerve (one of the main nerves to leg).

The reflex arc

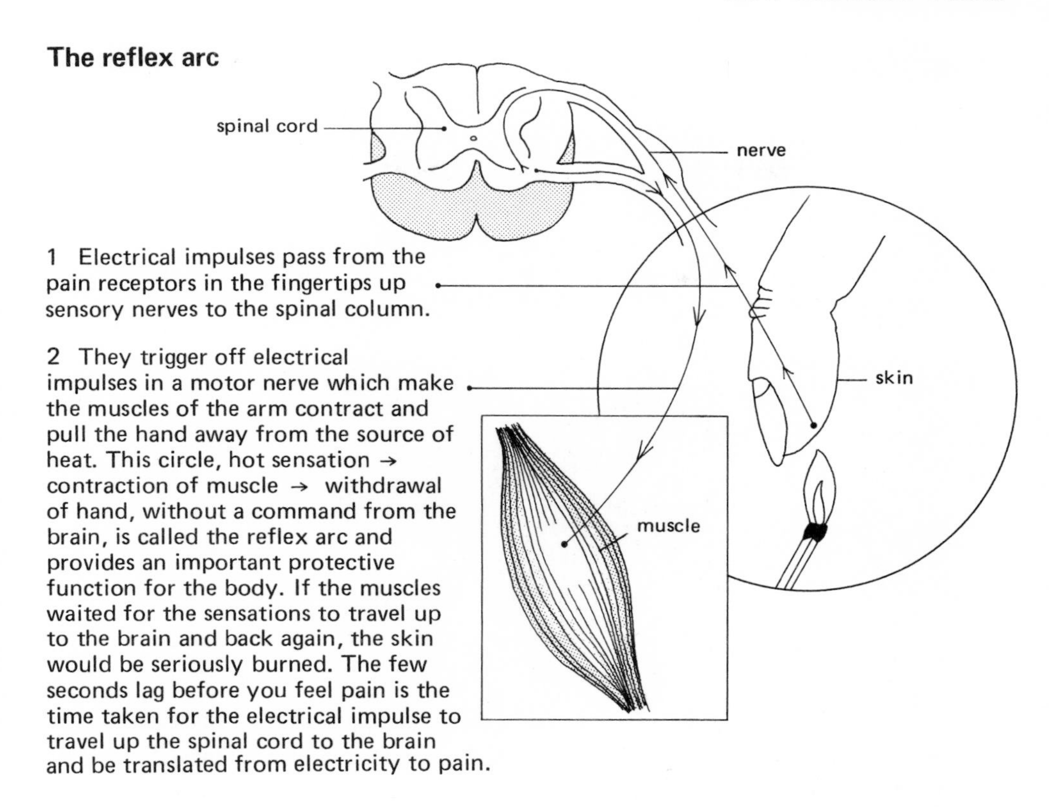

1 Electrical impulses pass from the pain receptors in the fingertips up sensory nerves to the spinal column.

2 They trigger off electrical impulses in a motor nerve which make the muscles of the arm contract and pull the hand away from the source of heat. This circle, hot sensation → contraction of muscle → withdrawal of hand, without a command from the brain, is called the reflex arc and provides an important protective function for the body. If the muscles waited for the sensations to travel up to the brain and back again, the skin would be seriously burned. The few seconds lag before you feel pain is the time taken for the electrical impulse to travel up the spinal cord to the brain and be translated from electricity to pain.

of the bladder and bowels, the movements of the stomach and intestines during digestion, and the regular contractions and relaxations of the diaphragm when we breathe. These nerve fibres congregate in the solar plexus and a severe blow to the abdomen can take your breath away so crippling is the internal pain. One part of the autonomic system prepares us for 'fight and flight' and the other part is for reparation, i.e. eating and sleeping. Interestingly sexual activity needs both parts.

The cardiovascular system

Your heart is about the size of your fist and not so different in shape. We tend to think of the heart as being on the left side of the chest, but it is more centrally placed with just the lower point of its triangle skewed to one side so that it is approximately in line with the left nipple.

The heart has four chambers; the upper ones are called atria and the two lower ones ventricles. Blood flows from top to bottom through the heart, entering the atria, passing down to the ventricles, and then out to the body. Blood from the right ventricle goes to the lungs and that from the left ventricle to the body.

Slice through the heart

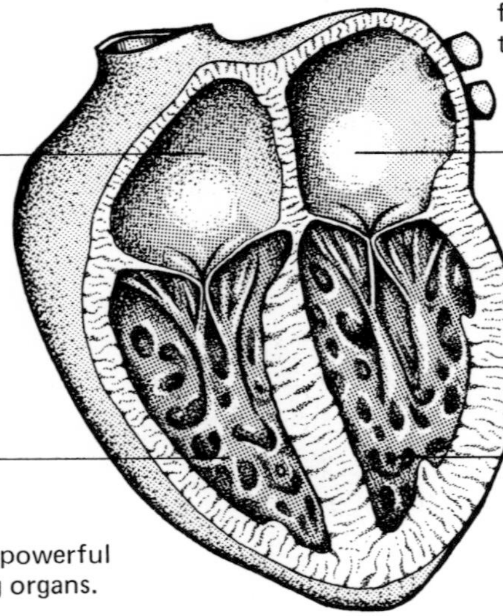

The atria are divided from the ventricles by valves. In health the valves are formed from two or three smooth shiny flaps which are opened and closed by very fine muscular strands from the wall of the heart itself.

The atria are really only reservoirs for the blood.

The ventricles are powerful muscular pumping organs.

The atrio-ventricular valves are one-way valves and when they close blood cannot regurgitate back into the atria. If the valves become diseased, as they may in rheumatic fever, so that they are stiff and cannot open fully, or are slack and allow leakage back, they cause heart 'murmurs'. When the doctor listens to your heart, instead of hearing the classical, well-defined 'lub-dub' heart sounds, he may find them obscured by a variety of blowing sounds or murmurs. Each murmur has a characteristic sound according to the valvular defect.

Think of the heart as being in two separate parts, a right and a left, because each side pumps blood synchronously to a different place.

The heart, arteries and veins form a complete circulatory system. With each beat, the heart pushes out a wave of blood which the doctor feels at your wrist when he takes your pulse. The head of pressure which is set up is the blood-pressure and this helps to keep the blood flowing back to the heart. The blood-pressure is measured as the number of millimetres of mercury it can support and has two components: the systolic pressure due to the great spurt of blood when the ventricles contract; and the diastolic pressure which is the 'holding' pressure. The blood pressure is described as the

systolic pressure/diastolic pressure; a normal blood-pressure is 120/80.

Increases in the systolic pressure are common and often transient; it rises in exercise, when we get excited and as we get older. The diastolic pressure is shifted much less easily and if it becomes permanently raised, it should be treated. A doctor would be concerned about a diastolic pressure of 95+ and a

The cardiovascular system

1 The right side of the heart receives blood, via the veins, which has been circulating round the body, and from which all the oxygen has been absorbed.

2 The right ventricle pumps the blood to the lungs where it takes up oxygen.

3 The veins of the lungs return the blood to the left side of the heart.

4 The newly oxygenated red blood is pumped through the main arteries to the most distant parts of the body.

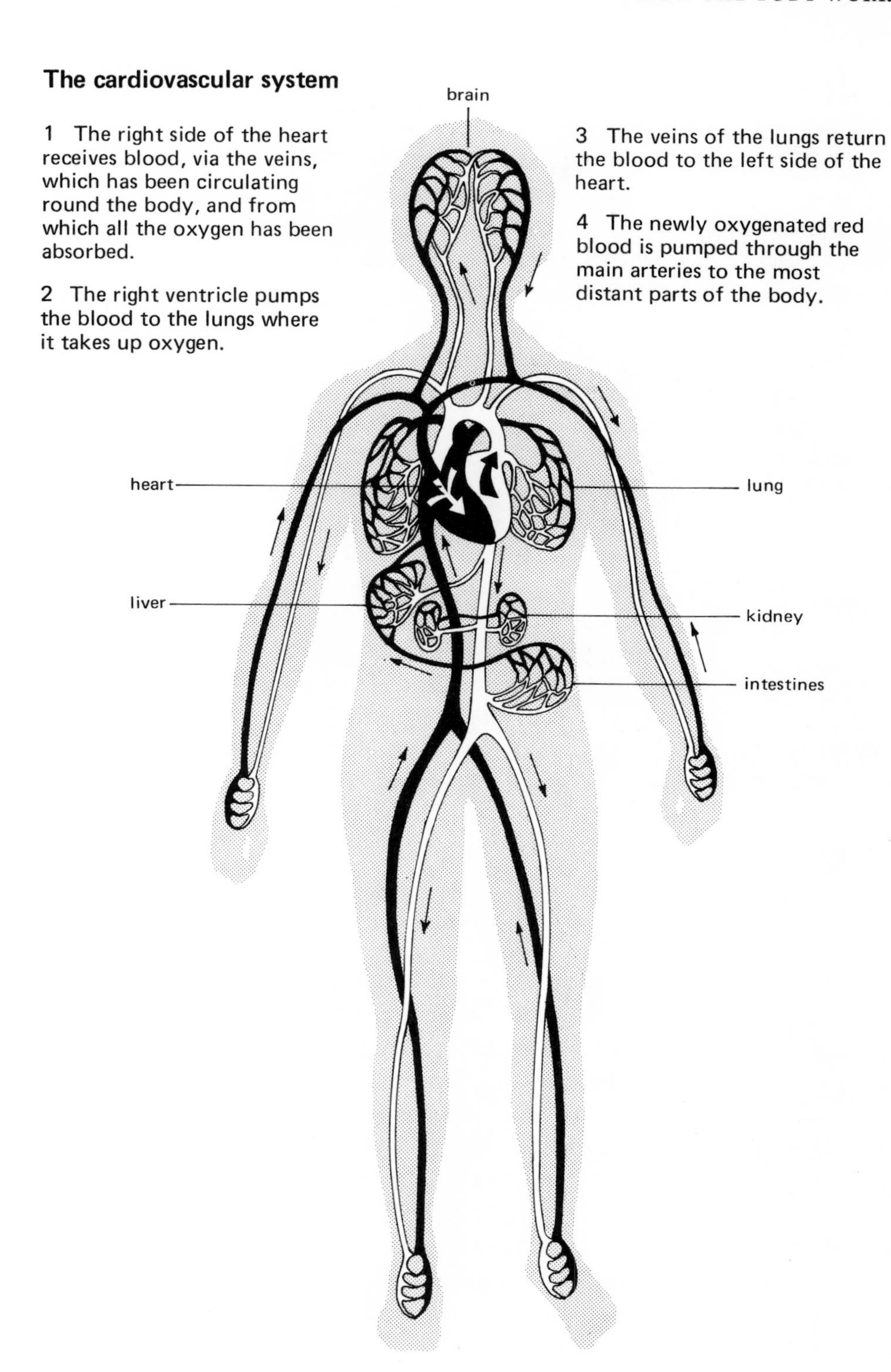

systolic of 150+ if present for any length of time. In pregnancy smaller increases, say 125/85, are treated immediately.

Coronary arteries supply the heart muscle. Death of the heart muscle, caused by the blockage of the coronary arteries, can lead to excruciating chest pain and collapse – myocardial infarction. Years before the blockage occurs the walls of the arteries are narrowed by fatty deposits. This can lead to angina, the pain from cardiac muscle which is not receiving sufficient oxygen from the trickle of blood flowing through the narrowed arteries.

Heart muscle is not the only muscle to produce crippling pain when deprived of oxygen. If you are prepared to repeat an experiment performed by most medical students you can experience it in your forearm. Bind your upper arm with a tight band and then start clenching and opening your fist. Because the blood-supply to your forearm is reduced to a fine stream by the constricting band, your hard-working muscles outstrip their oxygen supply and the pain becomes acute and unbearable in a short time. The pain is very similar in character to angina, the only difference being that the blood-supply to the heart is restricted by narrowed arteries, not by a tight band.

As arteries travel away from the heart, their branches become finer until finally they become capillaries with walls so thin that oxygen can pass through them into the tissues. Waste carbon dioxide diffuses into the capillaries from the tissues and is carried back to the right side of the heart for circulation through the lungs where it is released and expelled from the body when we exhale. A healthy heart can meet any demand from the body for more blood and in this way it plays one of its most important roles in helping to nourish the various parts of the body.

The lungs

In a healthy young person the lungs are two large, soft, spongy, pink bags filling most of the chest. In adults they are more often greyish-black from dust particles if we live in a smoky industrial area, or yellowish-brown from tars if we smoke more than ten cigarettes a day. One of the most important properties of the lungs is their elasticity. Within the housing of the semi-rigid rib cage, they stretch and contract during inhalation and exhalation forming, in conjunction with the diaphragm, an efficient bellows system. The diaphragm is a dome-shaped muscle which divides the chest from the abdomen and is attached to the ribs all the way round its circumference.

The lungs perform two very important functions for the body: they nourish the body with vital oxygen and they excrete waste carbon dioxide. Water is another waste product of metabolism and the air we exhale is full of moisture. So the lungs form part of our complex excretory system in tandem with the

The lungs and how they work

The right lung is divided into three lobes, upper, middle and lower, each of which receives a large branch from the main bronchus.
Because of the position of the heart, the left lung has only two lobes, both of which receive a large branch from the main bronchus.

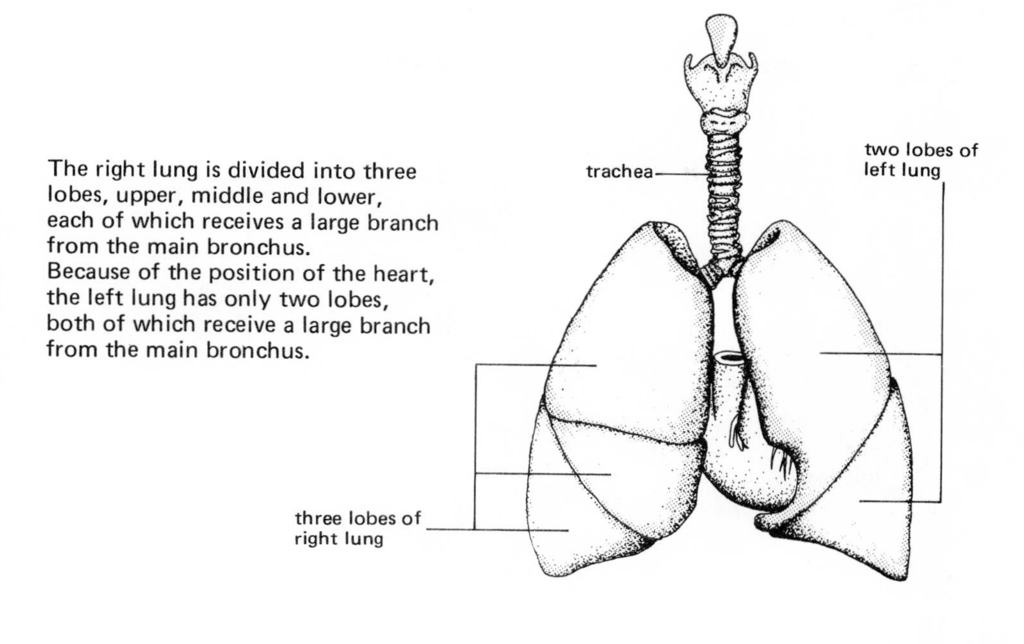

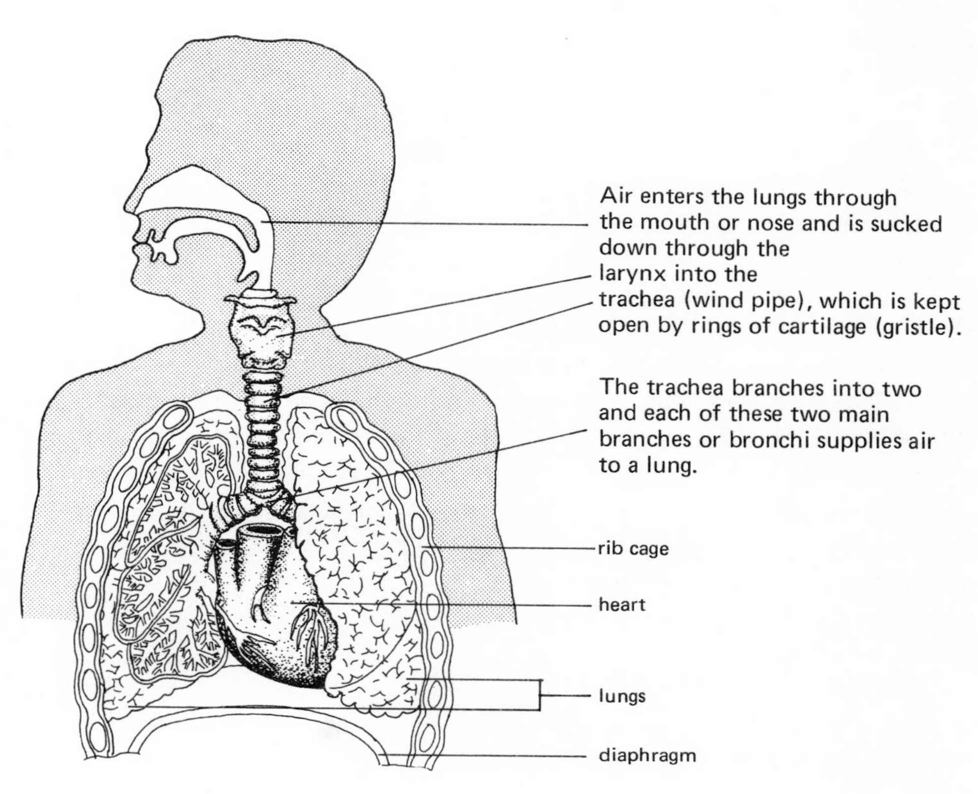

How the diaphragm works

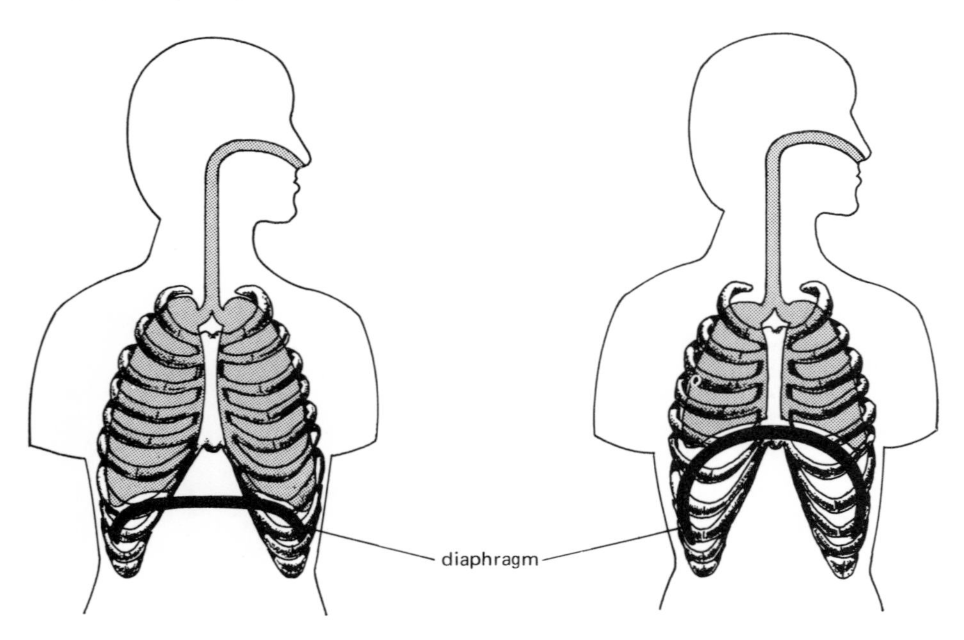

When the diaphragm contracts, the dome flattens out allowing the lungs to expand and take in air.

When the diaphragm relaxes, the dome rises and pushes up the lungs making us expire.

kidneys; the function of one perfectly complements the function of the other.

With this background you can understand what happens when the lungs are damaged. With bronchitis, the inflamed bronchi secrete an excess of mucus which we cough up and spit out. When a great deal of mucus is produced it will impede gaseous exchange between the air and blood by forming a lining round the membrane of the air sac. With an attack of asthma, the bronchi constrict to very narrow passages which gives the breathing a whistling note – wheezing. In these circumstances sufficient air can neither get in nor out of the lungs. The bellows break down. No matter how hard the diaphragm works, no matter how the ribs strive to move in and out, air simply cannot ventilate the lungs. Oxygen does not reach the air sacs to oxygenate the blood and turn it from 'blue' to 'red'. Gradually the 'blue' blood accumulates, which is why asthmatic people are cyanosed (have a bluish skin colour) during an attack.

The blood, spleen and lymphatic system

The blood is the fluid part of a single system composed of the spleen, the lymph glands and the bones. The connection between these different groups is

How the blood is oxygenated in the lungs

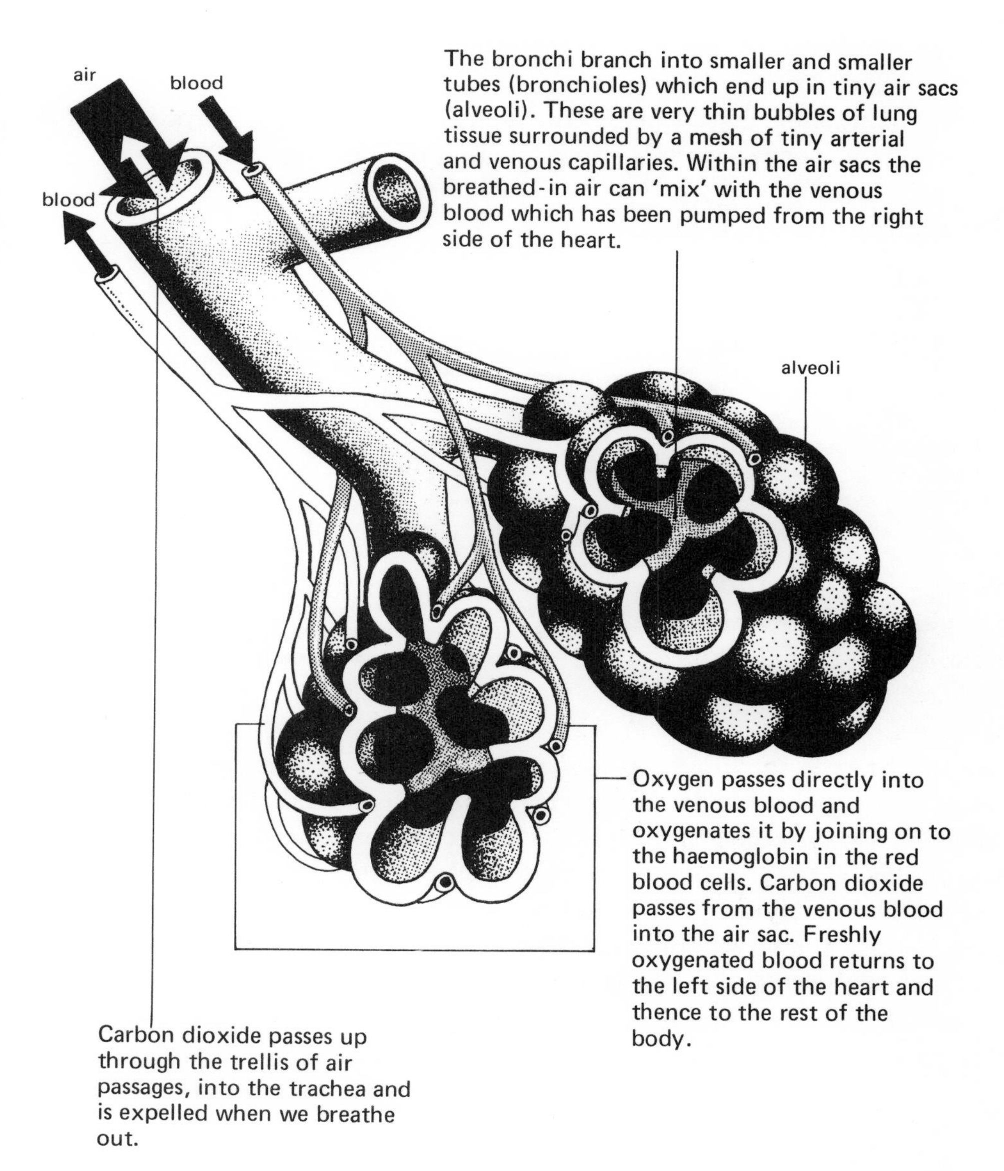

that the cells, like the red and white blood cells, are common to all of them. Furthermore, fluid is in a constant dynamic exchange between them.

Blood is initially manufactured by the bone marrow of the embryo. Bones such as the sternum (breast bone), the vertebrae and the limb bones are the factories for the blood cells, both red and white. In adults blood production is largely confined to the end of the long bones like the femur, the sternum and the bones of the pelvic girdle. Blood is constantly circulating through the bone marrow and new blood cells are quickly carried into the blood stream to do their crucial job as oxygen transporters (red cells) and defenders against infection (white cells).

The main components of blood are the disc-shaped red cells (corpuscles) and white cells suspended in clear straw-coloured plasma.

The composition of the blood

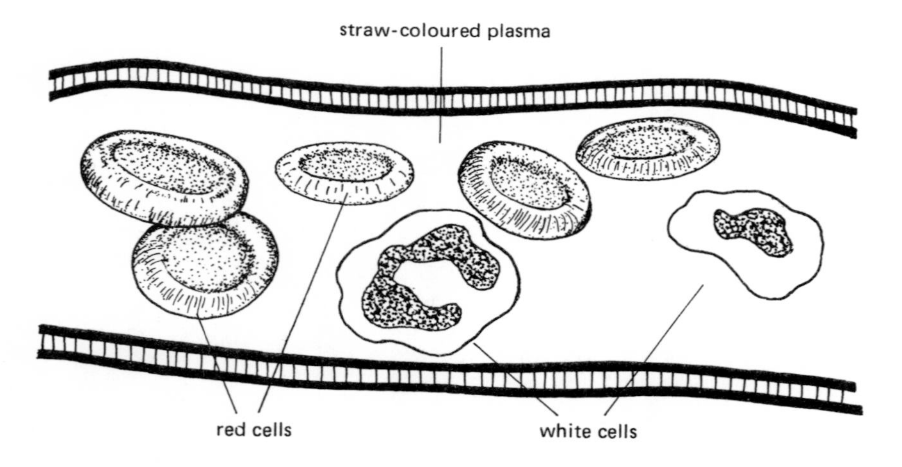

The red cells carry oxygen which is needed by all parts of the body to maintain crucial metabolic processes; without it, tissues die. Oxygen is chemically attached to haemoglobin, which is the red pigment in red blood cells and is responsible for the red colour of the blood. Haemoglobin is hungry for oxygen and will grab hold of it if there is plenty around. It will just as easily let go of oxygen when the surrounding need for it is great.

There are several kinds of white cell each with a specific part to play in defending the body. Some are mobile and migrate to a focus of infection where they engulf and destroy bacteria. Others help stave off the harmful effects of an allergic reaction. Yet others manufacture antibodies which paralyse bacteria and neutralize their poisons.

The spleen, which is situated just under the lower left side of the chest, is really a breakage and salvage depot for ageing blood cells. It filters off damaged or old (three- to four-month-old) blood cells, then breaks them up, returning useful material like iron to our body stores and getting rid of useless waste. The spleen also forms white blood cells – the kind that make antibodies.

The lymphatic system is a minor circulatory system where the fluid – almost transparent lymph – circulates round the body in membranous vessels. The system is subsidiary to the veins of the body and runs in parallel with them. Lymph is fluid which has seeped out of the blood vessels from the blood and drains into a gland or group of lymph glands, the most familiar of which are those in the tonsil area. If our tonsils become infected the lymph glands under the jaw often become sore and swollen because they are the first line in the body's defence against infection. They are acting as a filter system for bacteria and viruses, preventing them from penetrating other parts of the body. If you have an infection in your arm or leg you will find that the glands of the armpit or groin become swollen as they are performing the same watchdog function.

The liver

The liver, which lies under your rib cage on the right side of your body and weighs about three pounds, is intimately involved in many functions of the body from manufacturing proteins and antibodies to clotting of the blood and rendering poisons inactive. It acts as a purifying plant, as a storage organ and as a kind of chemical scrapyard. It has been called 'the chemical workshop of the body'.

The circulation of the blood from the stomach and the upper part of the intestine (the small, as opposed to the large, intestine) is so arranged that it passes through the liver first. Any poison or drug which is absorbed from the gut is partly filtered off by the liver and detoxicated (rendered harmless). The harmless by-products are excreted in the bile. The bile owes its greenish colour to the breakdown products of haemoglobin (the pigment in red blood cells). The breakdown products are transported through the liver by a system of tiny tubes to the main bile duct and stored in the gall bladder. Damage to liver cells or blockage in the bile ducts prevents normal elimination of bile. Bile pigment overflows into the blood and colours the skin and the conjunctivae of the eye yellow, i.e., jaundice.

Glycogen, a starch which is a rich source of energy, is stored in the liver. When the body needs energy the glycogen is rapidly split into sugar and released into the blood-stream.

The liver treats all unwanted chemicals in the same way whether they have come from the outside or, like hormones, are formed inside the body. Once they have done their job the liver turns the sex hormones, androgen, oestrogen and progesterone into inactive substances. The liver is crucial in protecting the body

Close-up of section through the liver

Inside the liver, bile and blood flow close together.

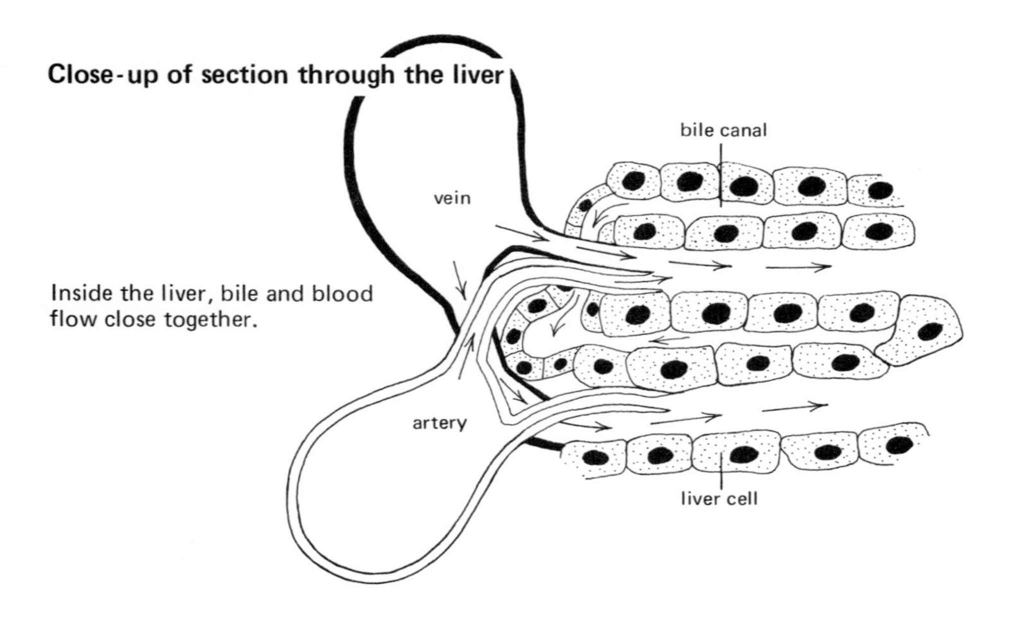

The liver and bile

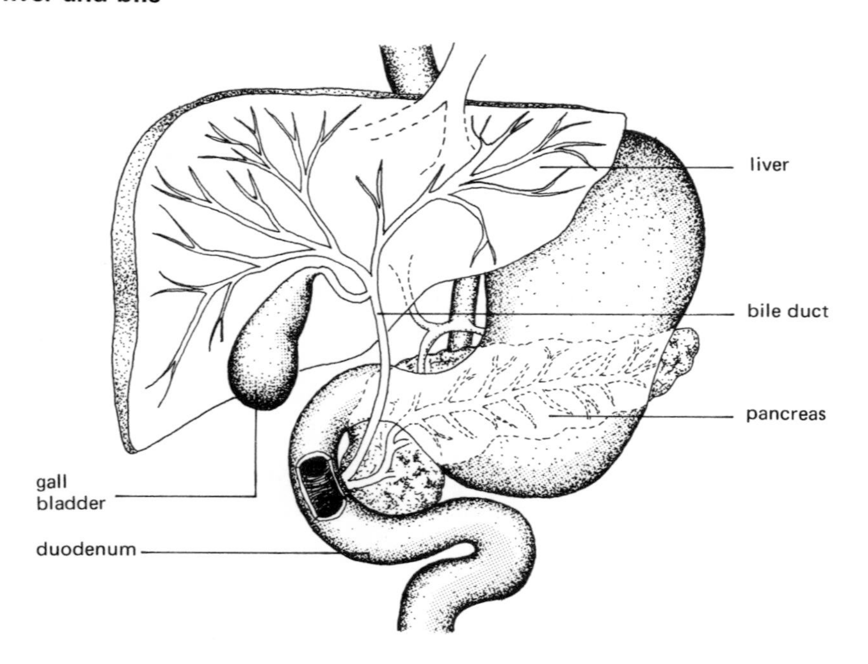

We make two pints of bile a day and it is stored in the gall bladder after leaving the liver.

The bile, which enters the duodenum through the bile duct, is necessary for the digestion of fats and is responsible for the brown colour of faeces.

against infection as it is a source of antibodies to infectious germs. It also synthesizes a substance called prothrombin which plays an important part in the clotting mechanism of the blood.

Alcohol is broken down in the liver. However, the liver can handle only so much and if alcohol is taken in too great a quantity it acts as a poison; liver cells are destroyed, the internal architecture of the liver becomes distorted and eventually it is unable to function properly. Liver failure ensues. Cirrhosis is the inevitable result of many years of hard drinking and, if not arrested, will eventually lead to coma and death.

The kidneys

Our two kidneys lie on either side of the spinal column and rest on the back of the ribs.

They are an integral part of our excretory system. Excretion is a specialized term referring to specific body processes; it is the production of waste products such as urine, sweat and carbon dioxide during metabolism within the body. Faeces are not a product of excretion because they are waste from food, not from internal metabolic reactions.

We make most urine during daylight hours and most of us have a surge first thing in the morning. During the night we secrete very little but urine from the night is much more concentrated and consequently more acid than that from the day. The main waste substance is urea which is the residue from the protein metabolism; it gives the urine most of its colour and smell.

We often talk about 'strong' urine which usually refers to its deep yellow colour or strong smell. The strength of urine depends mainly on the volume of

Slice through a kidney

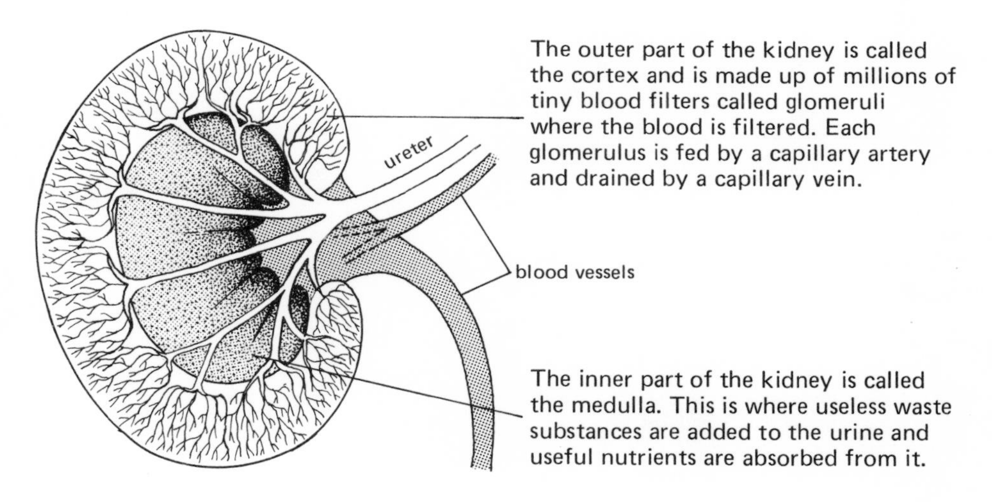

The urinary system

To filter the blood efficiently the kidneys have an excellent blood supply. There are large renal arteries and veins to the kidneys which split into very fine capillaries deep inside them.

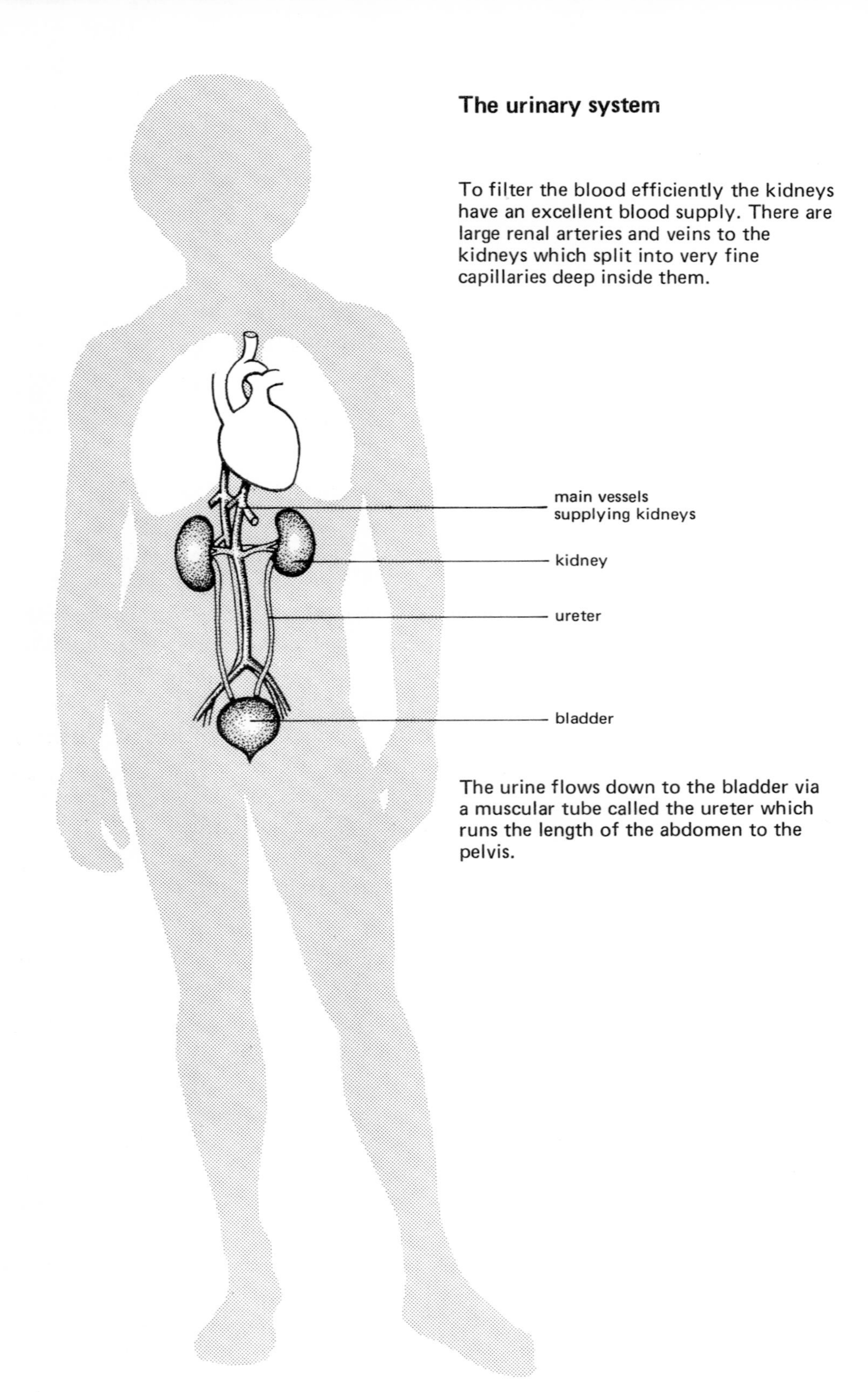

The urine flows down to the bladder via a muscular tube called the ureter which runs the length of the abdomen to the pelvis.

How the kidneys work

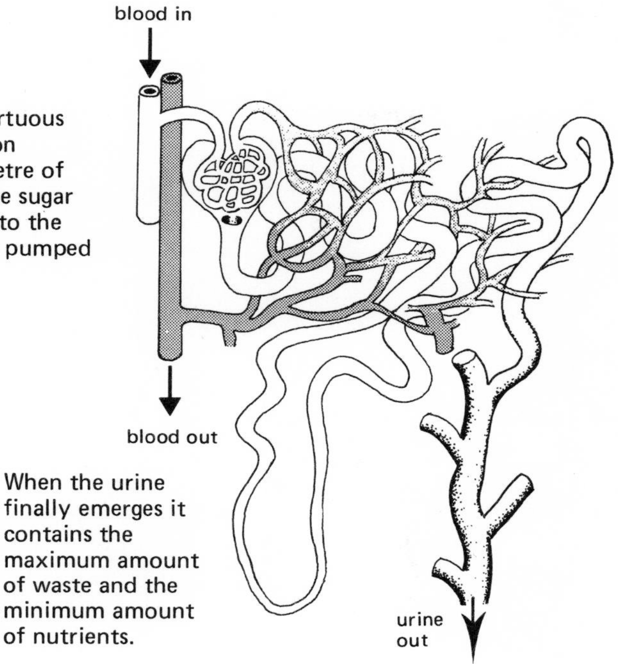

urine we produce – if the volume is small it will be strong and if the volume is large it will be weak. The volume we pass is dependent on how much fluid we drink; if we drink the suggested three and a half pints a day our urine will rarely be strong. However there is nothing wrong with strong urine since it rarely denotes anything more than a low fluid intake and indeed is a sign that the kidneys are functioning properly. Many substances appear in the urine within a short time of ingesting them; for example, urine may become pinkish a few hours after eating beetroot and you can smell ampicillin (an antibiotic related to penicillin) in the urine thirty minutes after swallowing a capsule. Many people have been frightened by the blackish urine they pass after eating liquorice.

The gastro-intestinal tract

You can think of the gastro-intestinal tract as a tube which runs right through the middle of the body but which, in a very real sense, is not 'inside' it. The mouth and anus are the openings at either end of the tube. Food enters through the mouth and, as though on a conveyor belt, has various things added to and removed from it. It finally emerges through the anus as faeces without ever having really 'entered' the body.

All the different chemical and enzymatic reactions that take place in the gastro-intestinal tract are leading to one thing – the breakdown of complex food

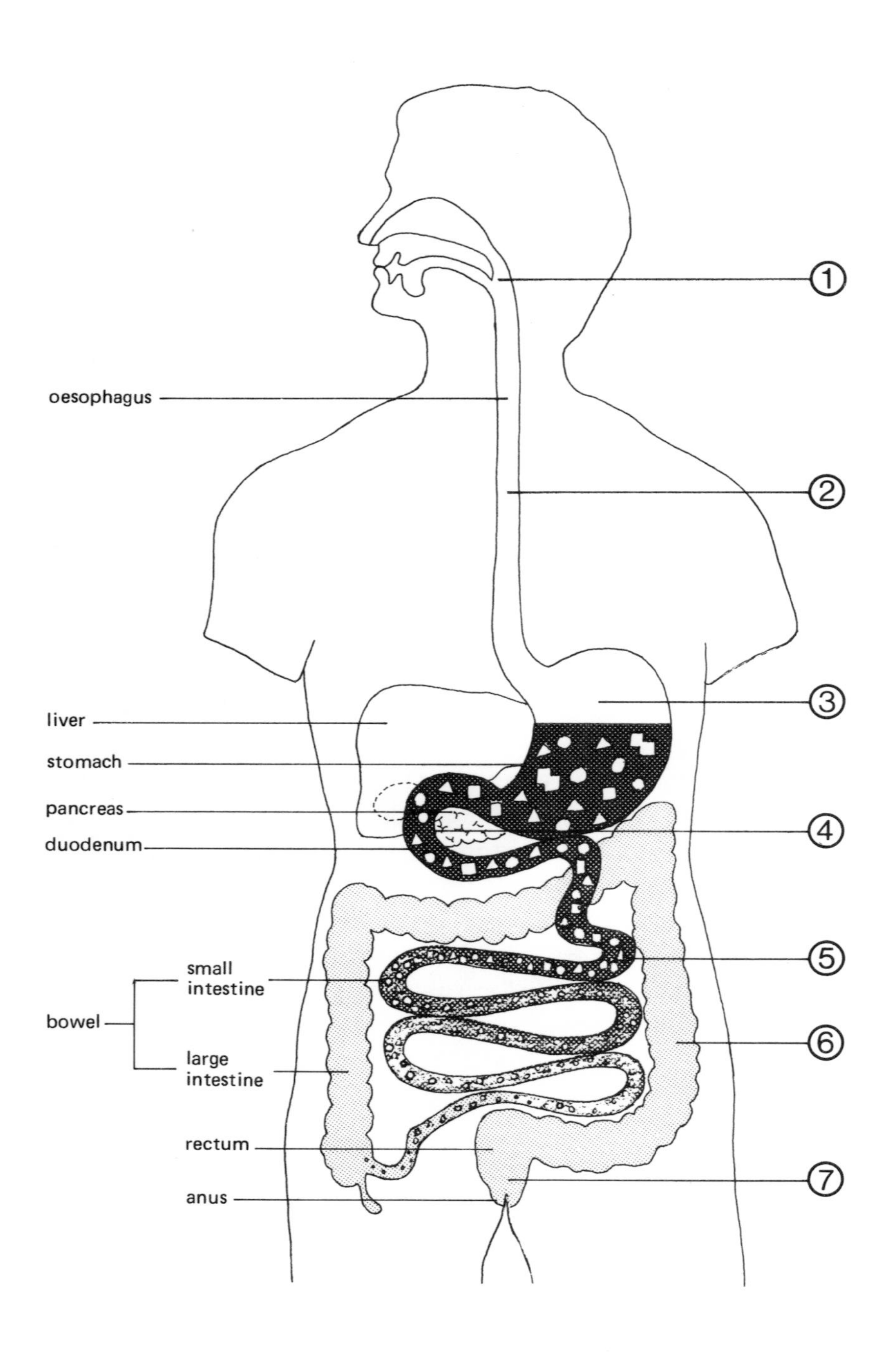

1
oesophagus
2
3
liver
stomach
pancreas
4
duodenum
5
small
intestine
bowel
6
large
intestine
rectum
7
anus

How food passes through the body

1 In the mouth food is ground into a semi-solid pulp which is swallowable. It becomes mixed with saliva which contains an enzyme that acts on certain starchy foods. Thus the digestive process begins with our first chew.

2 Swallowed food passes into the oesophagus (gullet) and is pushed down towards the stomach by ripples of muscular contractions.

3 The stomach is a grinding, storage and digestive organ. In it the food is mixed with fairly strong hydrochloric acid which is necessary for the enzymatic action of pepsin on protein foods. Pepsin is a proteolytic enzyme, i.e. it breaks down large protein molecules into smaller-sized particles. When the contents of the stomach are mixed to a fine sludge they are fed out in small quantities into the duodenum. The duodenum (and the oesophagus) are unprotected against the acidity of the stomach which is why an excess of acid in the stomach leads to peptic ulceration.

4 In the duodenum the food becomes alkaline and enzymes from the pancreas and bile from the gall bladder are mixed with it to complete digestion of starches, proteins and fats.

5 Most of the proteins, fats, vitamins and minerals in our food are absorbed further down the small intestine where the surface area of the gut is greatly increased by many microscopic finger-like projections.

6 In the large intestine much of the water is absorbed from the food, converting it to solid faeces. If food is hurried through too quickly, for example with a bowel infection, then water cannot be absorbed and the stool becomes very liquid, i.e. diarrhoea.

7 Faeces emerge without ever having really 'entered' the body. The rectum conveniently does not have to empty itself continuously, but usually responds to the entrance of food into the stomach with the 'call to stool'. This reflex is known as the gastro-colic reflex and ignoring it is one of the commonest causes of constipation.

Vital organs of the digestive system

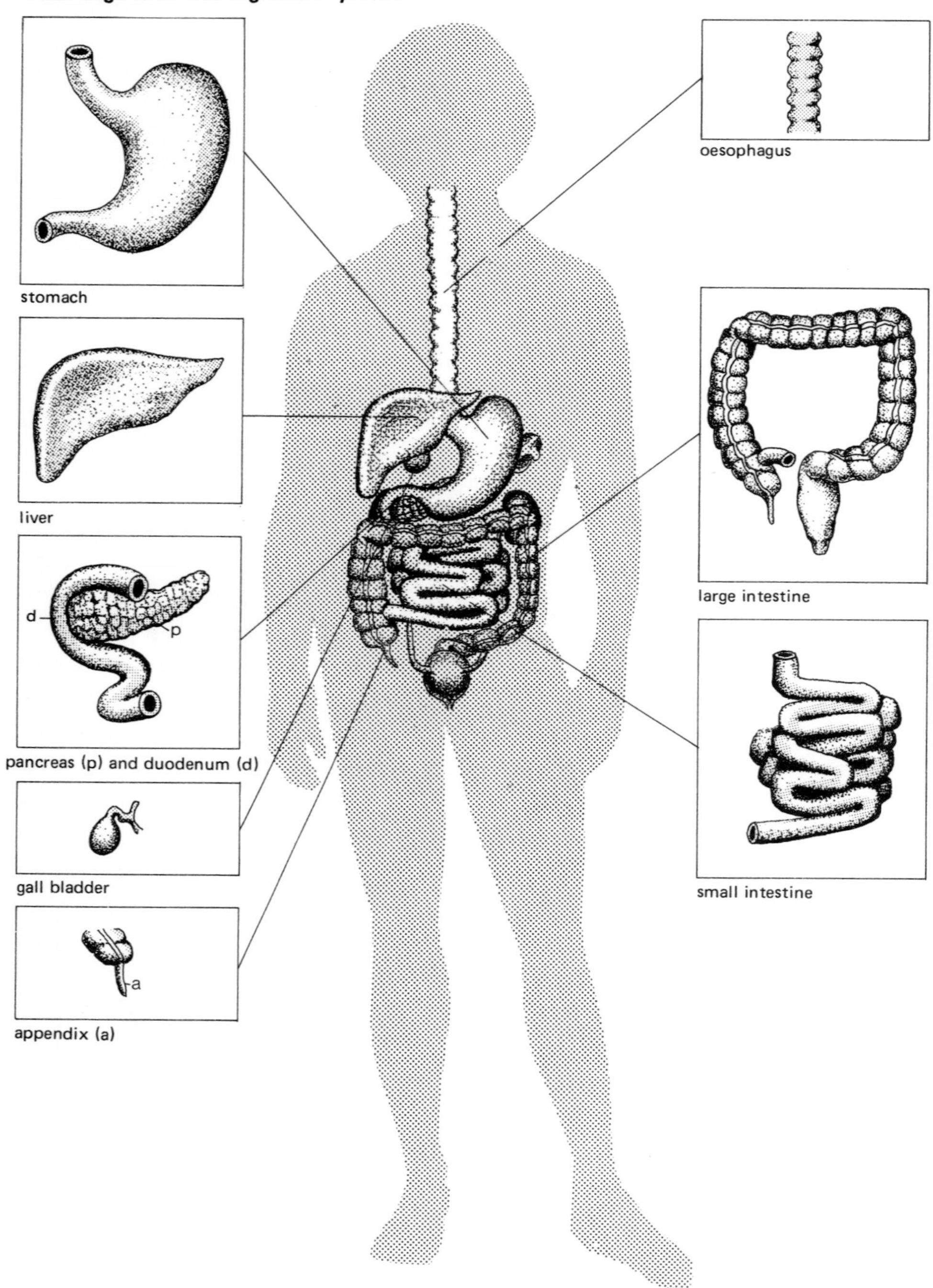

stomach

liver

pancreas (p) and duodenum (d)

gall bladder

appendix (a)

oesophagus

large intestine

small intestine

molecules into small enough moieties to pass through the wall of the intestine and into the blood-stream in order to nourish us. To this end there are mechanical grinders like teeth and muscular churners like the stomach; there are chemical disintegrators, enzymes, secreted by the stomach and duodenum, which split up large complicated chemical molecules into small simple ones; and, finally, there are digestive solvents or juices which will dissolve small chemical molecules into solution, thereby facilitating their absorption in the intestine.

The endocrine (hormone glands) system

The hormone glands are responsible for a system of chemical messengers which are manufactured in one part of the body, enter the blood and are carried to another part of the body where they exert their effect. To demonstrate how this system works, let us take adrenalin as an example. If we feel frightened, the sensation of fear causes an increase in adrenalin output from the adrenal glands. Adrenalin constricts the blood-vessels in the skin (we go pale) and diverts all the blood to our muscles ready for flight. It also stimulates the heart to beat faster and more strongly. As fear subsides, so does the amount of adrenalin pouring into the blood. The heart slows and, as the muscles no longer need a lot of blood, the vessels in the skin open up and the colour comes back to our cheeks.

There are several simple endocrine glands that are making hormones which exert different effects on various parts of the body. These glands act only as team members and, as you might expect, there is a team leader – the pituitary gland in the brain – which has the job of secreting control hormones that stimulate the secretion of specific hormones. For instance, the pituitary secretes a control hormone ACTH, which stimulates the adrenal cortex to produce cortisone (the main life-giving hormone). Similarly, the thyroid is stimulated by a hormone secreted in the brain, as are the ovaries and the testes.

The brain, the pituitary, each gland and its hormone act together through a mechanism called 'negative feedback'. It is rather similar to the way in which blood sugar is controlled by insulin (see page 12). If the levels of androgens in the circulating blood fall, the brain produces more testicular-stimulating hormones which stimulate the testes to secrete more of their own hormone. When this pours into the blood, the brain picks up the message and switches off the production of testicular-stimulating hormone.

By this very delicate see-saw effect the various hormones circulating within the blood are held at just the right levels. Think of the hormone glands as members of an orchestra with the brain as the conductor; together they play in perfect rhythm and harmony.

The endocrine system

The pituitary gland secretes hormones affecting other endocrine glands, e.g. thyroid-stimulating hormone, and also milk secretion and growth.

The thyroid gland makes thyroid hormone which affects growth and the metabolic rate.

The parathyroid glands make parathyroid hormone which affects the amount of calcium and phosphorus in the body and the bones.

The adrenal glands (situated on the upper poles of the kidneys) have a medulla producing adrenalin and a cortex which secretes steroids, affecting most aspects of metabolism within the body.

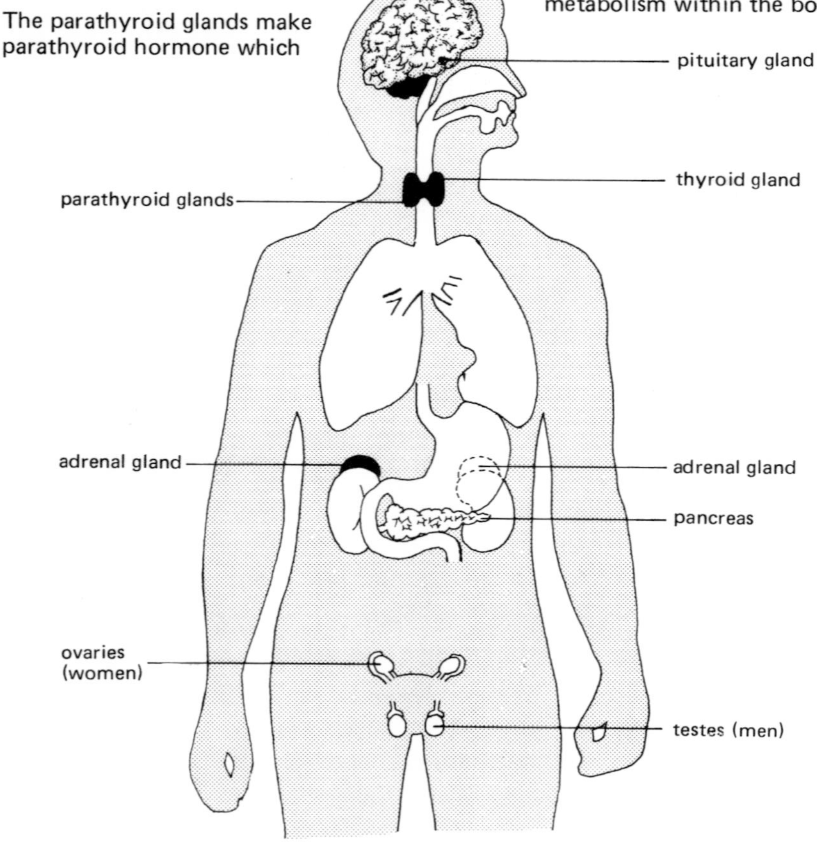

Insulin is secreted by the pancreas and lowers the blood sugar.

The ovaries secrete oestrogen and progestogen which affect the endometrium (the lining of the womb), the breasts and maintain a healthy pregnancy.

The testes manufacture androgens (male hormones) which are responsible for the characteristics of men.

The reproductive organs

The reproductive organs are, from one point of view, the most important since without them the human race would perish. In both sexes they are of two types – the genital organs and the sex-hormone glands.

In females the hormone glands are the two ovaries which alternately drop an egg in the middle of every menstrual cycle for the whole of a woman's fertile years. In the first half of the cycle the ovary produces oestrogen, and in the second half a mixture of oestrogen and progesterone. The changing levels of these hormones cause the monthly shedding of the endometrium, the lining of the womb, and thus the menstrual period. At puberty the levels rise steeply. This rise leads to the development of physical characteristics of the female, such as breasts and feminine contours.

The male hormone glands are the testes which secrete testosterone. Testo-

How the level of female hormones in the blood is controlled

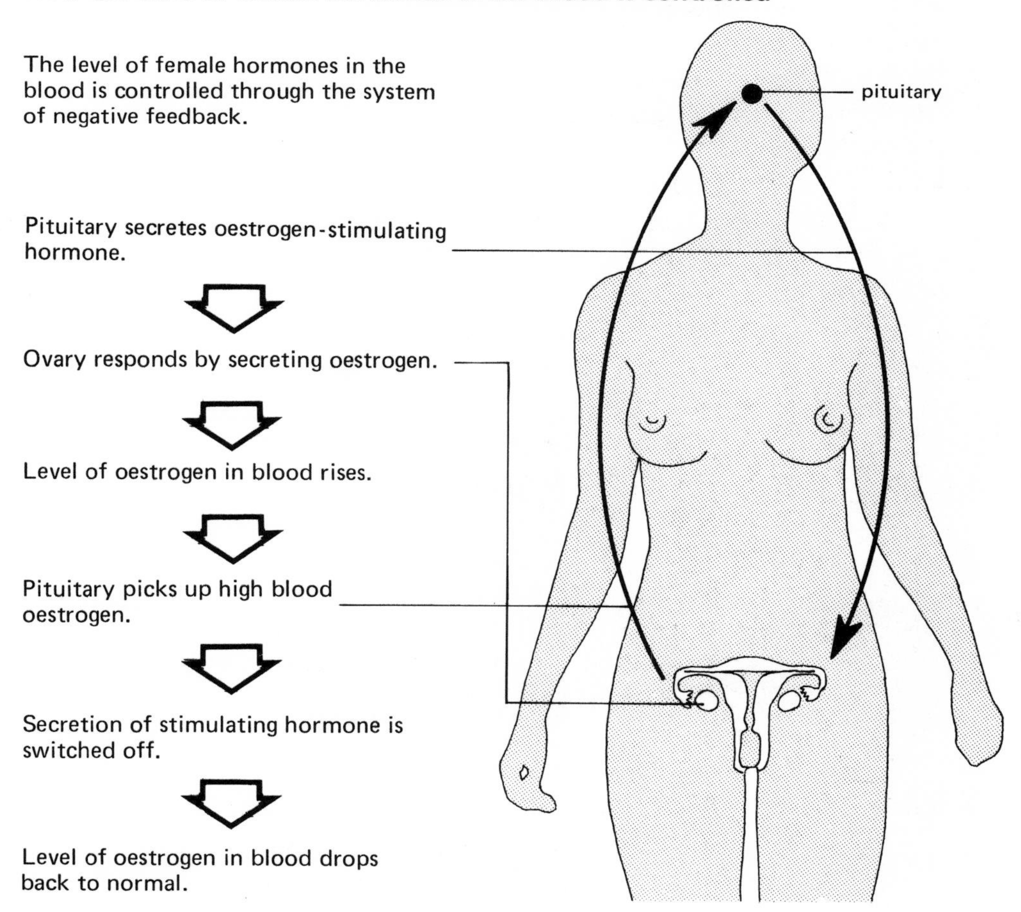

How the level of male hormones in the blood is controlled

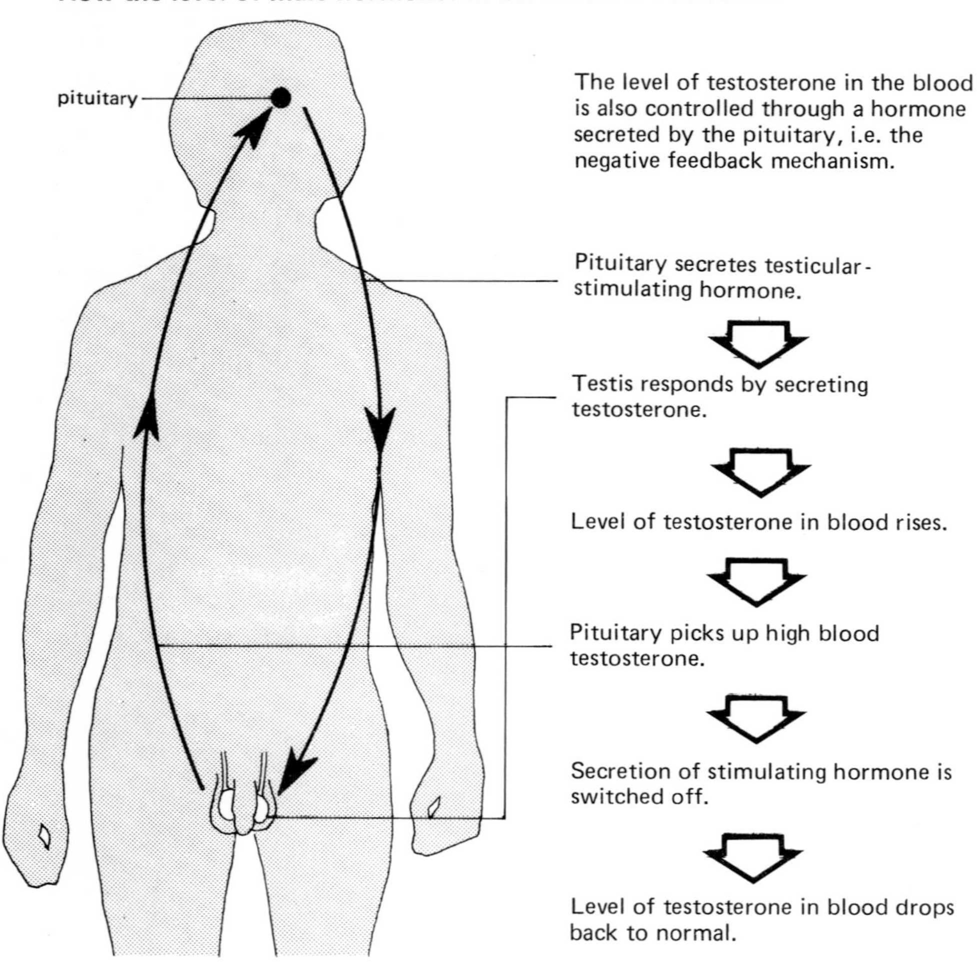

sterone causes male body characteristics like lowering of the voice, growth of the beard and hair on the chest, broad shoulders, narrow waist and large muscles and bones. It is also responsible for much of the drive in men – their more aggressive instincts such as ambition and competitiveness. The other function of the testes is to produce sperm continuously. Although men are not subject to regular monthly cycles like women, it is thought that the secretion of testosterone may follow several shorter cycles, weekly or even daily.

The sensory system

The sensory system relays messages from the outside world to the brain through seeing, hearing, smelling, tasting, touching and balancing. Compared to some other members of the animal kingdom our system is grossly inferior; we cannot see as well as the eagle, we cannot hear as well as most wild animals, we cannot smell as well as the dog, and our sense of balance is not as acute as a cat's. In one area, however, our sensory system is superior to any found in the animal world: the skin of our fingertips contains thousands of sensory organs which perceive and relay to the brain the feelings of hot, cold, pain and touch. This high degree of tactile sophistication is responsible for our manual dexterity and makes us unique among all animals. Nowhere but in the fingertips is there such a concentration of sensory glands. You can demonstrate this for yourself by a simple experiment. Prick a pin repeatedly into your fingertips and you will find that there is no spot you can prick without feeling it. Now get someone to prick a less sensitive area, such as your back. There may be an inch and a half between painful pinpricks so sparse are the pain receptors.

Messages from the eye reach the brain more quickly than those from the inner ear, which involve the flow of a viscous liquid (see p. 37). When these messages are in conflict we may feel sick as in seasickness. If the sea is choppy, the movements of the deck, the boat, the sea and the horizon are transmitted to the brain faster by our eyes than by our ears. By the time the message from the inner ear reaches the brain, the eyes are sending a different message to the brain.

The eye

The eye enables us to see by treating light in two stages:

1 The lens bends rays of light so that we can focus on objects.

2 The retina changes light rays into electrical impulses which the brain can translate into visual images.

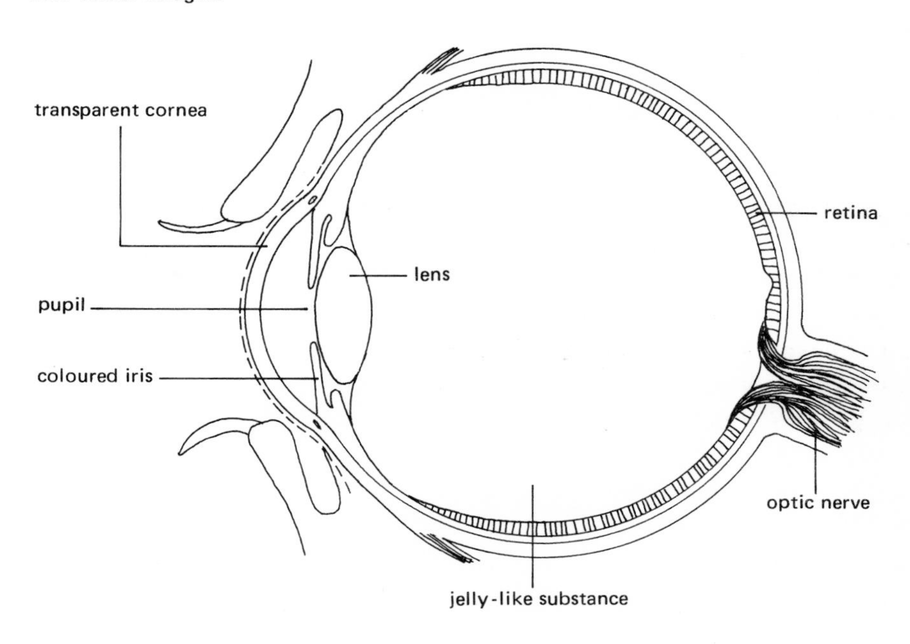

How we see

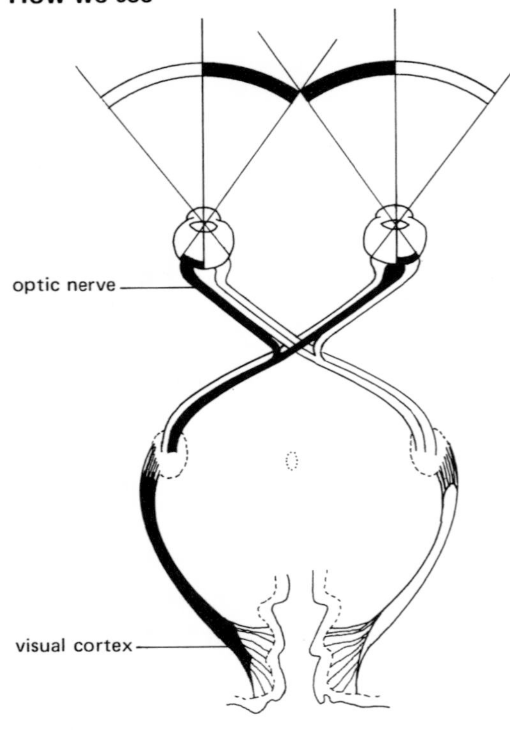

1 Light rays from the object we are looking at enter the eye and are focused on the retina by the lens, which will fatten or elongate according to whether the object is near or far away. Because the light rays cross before impinging on the retina the image is upside down.

2 Electrical impulses pass along the optic nerve to the visual cortex of the brain which is at the back of the head. By the time the image reaches the visual cortex it has been partly inverted and the brain completes the job of perceiving it the right way up.

Thus the brain receives conflicting information about the position of the body in relation to its surroundings; it becomes so confused that we feel dizzy and may quite often be sick.

The musculo-skeletal system

The musculo-skeletal system is composed of bones, muscles and joints. Bones form the skeleton, the joints between the bones make it moveable, and muscles move it.

The bones form the rigid, enormously strong girders on which the rest of our body is slung. They provide attachments for muscles without which our rather inflexible skeleton would be immobile. They are also protective: in the case of the chest and ribs, they protect the soft tissue of the lungs; in the case of the pelvic girdle, they protect the bladder, the gut and other internal organs. The bones make up much of the body's weight and strength. Male bones are always larger, thicker and stronger than female bones; on average, women will never be taller, heavier or stronger than men.

Muscles contain an elastic protein, myoglobin, which can shorten and lengthen when stimulated by motor nerves. When muscles shorten they usually

How the ear works

Functionally the ear can be divided into three parts:
1 The outer ear or pinna which focuses sound waves on to the eardrum.
2 The middle ear which hears.
3 The inner ear which contains the organ of balance.

1 The outer ear consists of the lobe and the external canal and ends at the eardrum.

2 We hear sounds with the middle ear. Sound waves impinge on the eardrum and make it vibrate. These vibrations are transmitted via a chain of three tiny bones, the 'stirrup', 'anvil' and 'hammer' bones, the so-called 'auditory ossicles', to sensitive nerve endings in the cochlea. In the nerve endings, sound waves are converted to electrical impulses and the sound is conducted to the auditory cortex of the brain where it is perceived as true sound. The middle ear is connected to the throat by the Eustachian tube which keeps the air pressure equal on either side of the eardrum. When it is blocked (e.g., during a cold) or if the air pressure changes too fast for the air to get up the tube (e.g., in an aeroplane) our ears pop.

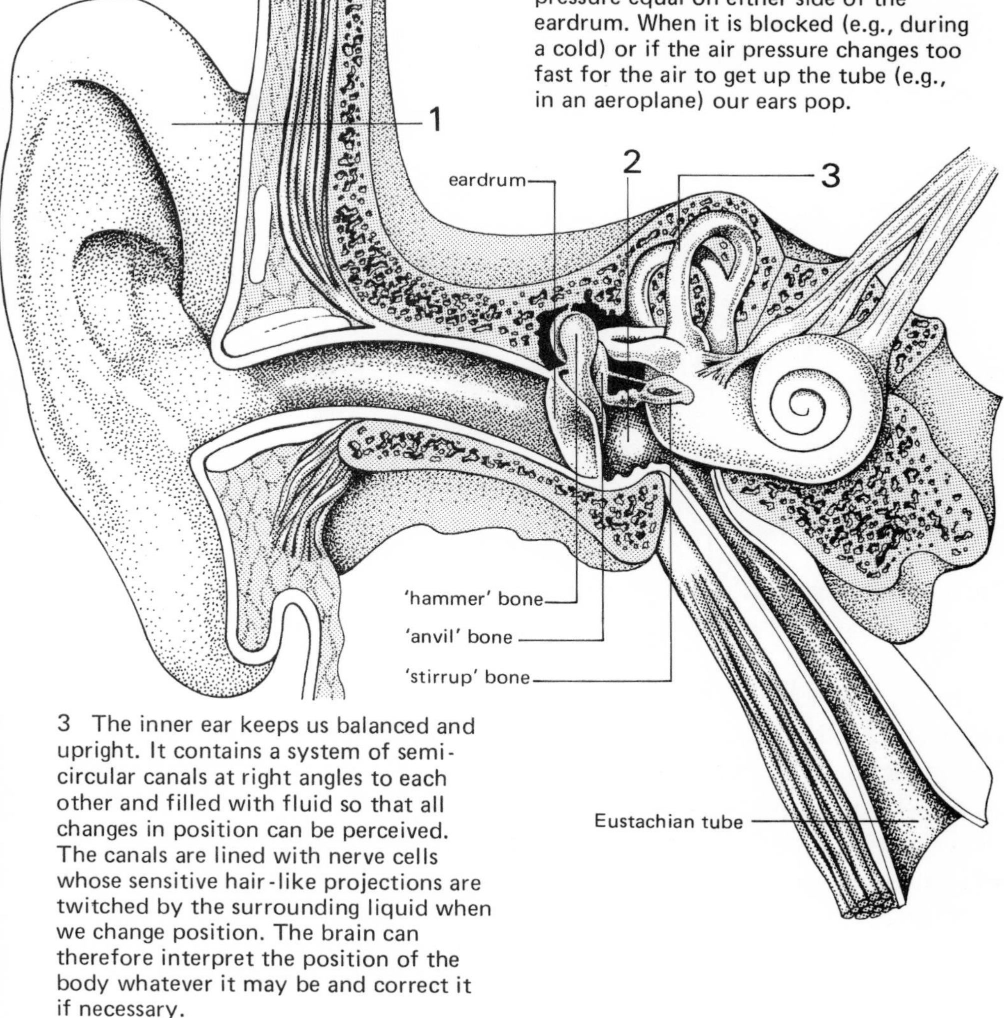

3 The inner ear keeps us balanced and upright. It contains a system of semicircular canals at right angles to each other and filled with fluid so that all changes in position can be perceived. The canals are lined with nerve cells whose sensitive hair-like projections are twitched by the surrounding liquid when we change position. The brain can therefore interpret the position of the body whatever it may be and correct it if necessary.

The skeleton

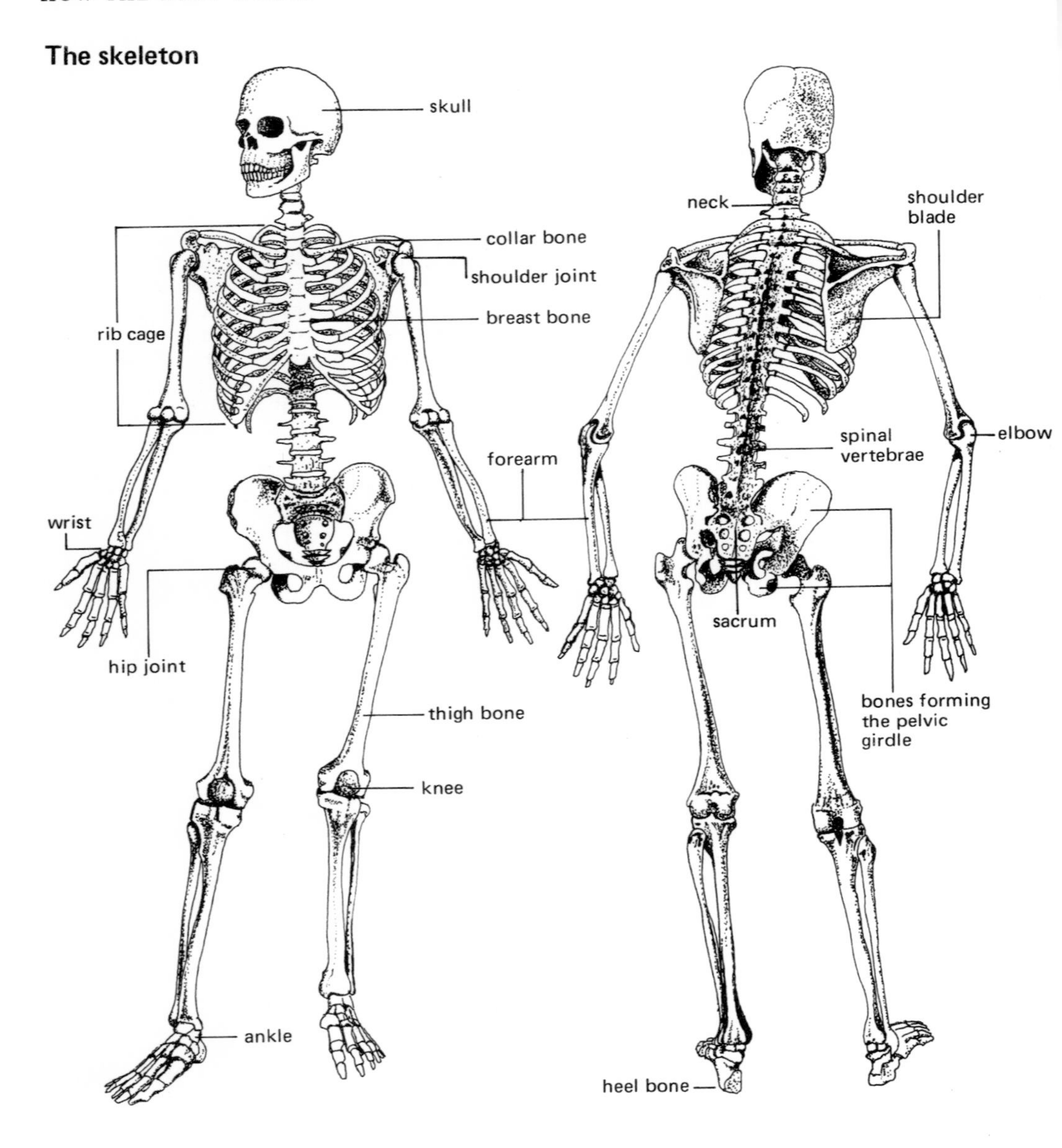

bend a joint, and when they relax the joint can straighten out again. Muscles are usually found in 'groups' which perform specific movements by working together – for instance, the muscles of the upper arm.

Our musculo-skeletal system owes its versatility of movement to the exquisite engineering of our joints; they are almost frictionless. It is only when joints become old and gritty, or inflamed, swollen and painful that we become aware of them. When the cartilage loses its shine and becomes rough and the synovial fluid becomes slightly thicker than normal, every movement of the joint causes pain: this is arthritis.

How the muscles of the upper arm work

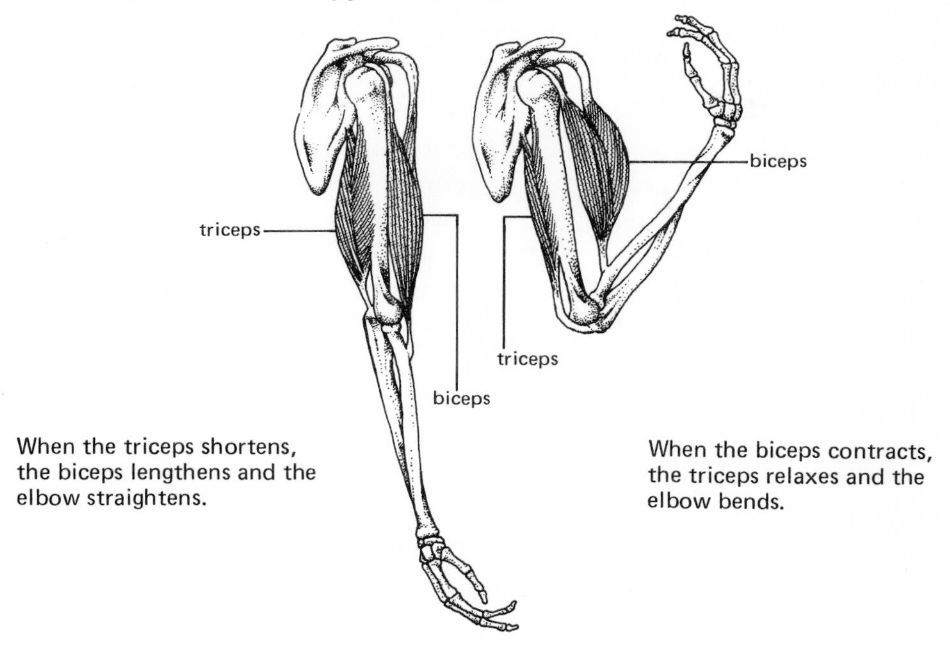

When the triceps shortens, the biceps lengthens and the elbow straightens.

When the biceps contracts, the triceps relaxes and the elbow bends.

How joints work

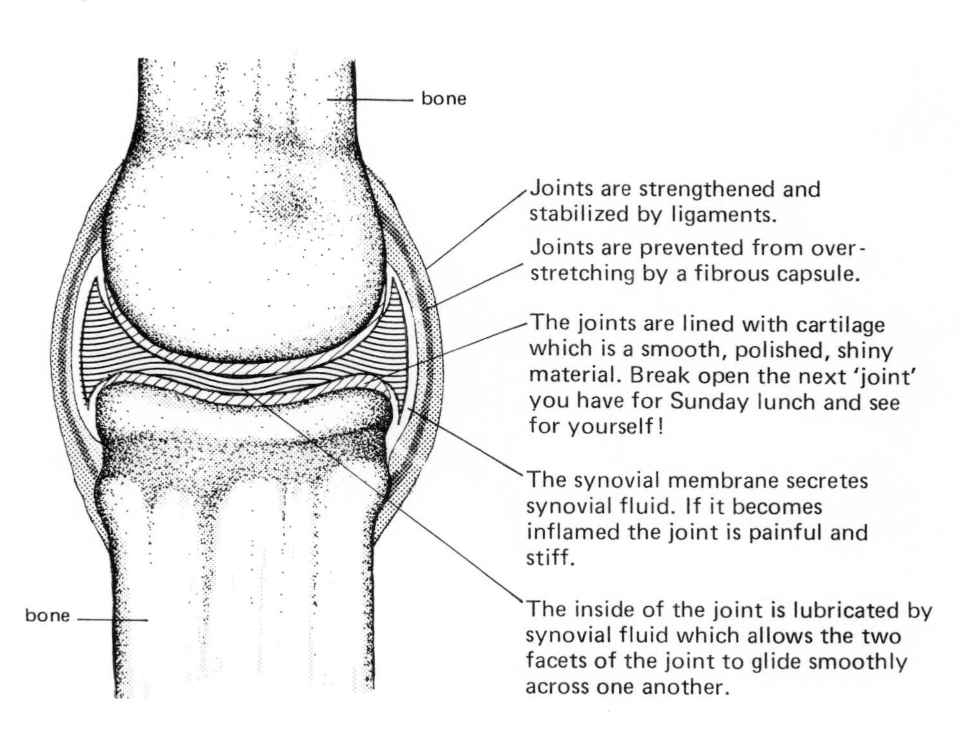

The skin

The skin is the largest organ of the body and performs several vital functions: it forms an efficient barrier to noxious agents and is relatively impermeable to weak acids and alkalis; it produces its own antiseptics which form an 'acid mantle' discouraging bacterial growth; and it maintains the body temperature. The skin maintains homeothermy by controlling the amount of sweat we produce and therefore the amount of heat we lose by evaporation; by opening up the blood-vessels in the skin to allow blood to lose heat to the cool surrounding air; and by flattening the body hair so that the layer of insulating air which normally stops heat loss and keeps the body warm is no longer trapped near the skin.

The skin is a living organ and is constantly replacing itself from within. New cells grow up from the living layer of the epidermis, mature, die and are shed from the surface in their hundreds of thousands every day. If the dead cells are in any way prevented from being shed, e.g. by the hair, they quickly pile up and form scales, e.g. dandruff.

The skin

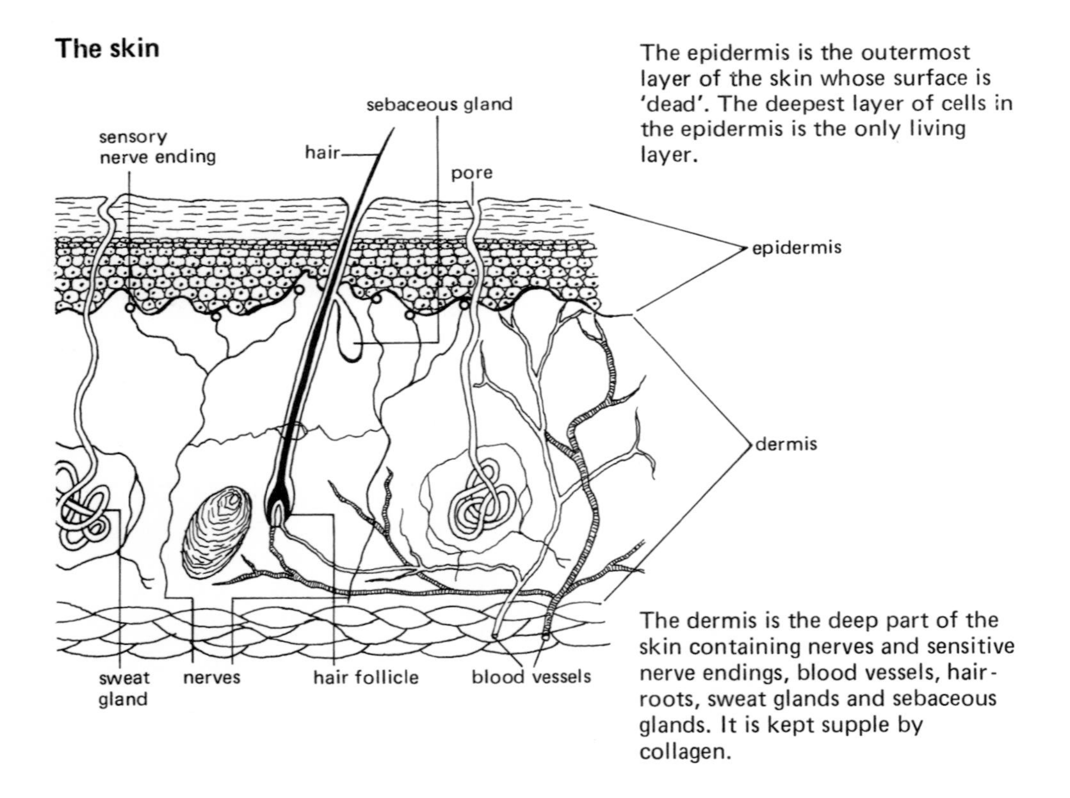

The epidermis is the outermost layer of the skin whose surface is 'dead'. The deepest layer of cells in the epidermis is the only living layer.

The dermis is the deep part of the skin containing nerves and sensitive nerve endings, blood vessels, hair-roots, sweat glands and sebaceous glands. It is kept supple by collagen.

2 The Importance of Diet

In western society we are overfed and overnourished. We are hardly ever hungry. Our days are punctuated by feeding and most of us eat fairly late at night. This is contrary to the way our bodies were designed to function. Animals can run faster and further when their stomachs are empty, and in the days when we were hunters this superior performance when we were hungry contributed to our survival. Athletes never undertake strenuous exercise within a short time of taking food, and most examination candidates will tell you they get better results if they take the exam on an empty stomach. Yet we live in an almost constant state of repletion, a state which was probably unknown to our ancestors whose lives were geared to intermittent hunger. The amount we eat and the kind of food we eat is almost certainly related to some of the killer diseases of our time.

There is a tribe living in northern Mexico among whom death from cardiac or circulatory disease is totally unknown. These people are thin and small and weigh on average less than nine and a half stone. Their daily calorie intake is well below the level recommended by the nutritional experts in developed countries who say the Mexicans are undernourished. These people can run races lasting a continuous forty-eight hours while maintaining a steady pace of six miles an hour for over 150 miles. They chase deer until the animals drop from exhaustion. Could it be that the western nutritionists are wrong and that these Mexicans are ideally nourished and we are overnourished? There is no doubt that most of us eat a great deal more than we *need*.

While almost every magazine we pick up has something to say about diet, calories and nutrition, the basic truths are very simple. To be healthy we need water, vitamins, minerals, protein and calories.

Vitamins and minerals

Despite the fact that we are a society obsessed with vitamins, it is unnecessary to give detailed information on the number of units each of us needs at different times of our lives of the vitamins A to K, including twelve forms of vitamin B not to mention the number of micrograms, milligrams or grams of calcium, phosphorus, manganese and other essential minerals. The fact is that no one in the western world who eats the balanced diet that is available to all of us,

Foods which are good sources of vitamins and minerals

Vitamin	Food
A (retinol)	Liver, milk, butter, eggs, tomatoes, carrots.
B_1 (thiamine)	Lean meat, especially pork, milk, wholewheat, brown rice.
B_2 (riboflavin)	Milk, cheese, liver, yeast, eggs, chicken.
B_6 (pyridoxine)	Liver, yeast, potatoes (especially in the skin).
Biotin	Peanuts, yeast.
Niacin (nicotinic acid)	Potatoes, fish, meat, peanuts, wholewheat.
B_3 (pantothenic acid)	Beans, cereals, liver.
Folic acid	Yeast, green vegetables.
B_{12} (cyanocobolamin)	Milk, eggs, fish, liver.
C (ascorbic acid)	Fresh fruit, especially citrus fruits, and vegetables, especially tomatoes.
D (calciferol)	Fish oils, milk, butter, margarine. Sunshine activates it in skin.
K	Liver, green vegetables, tomatoes.
Iron	Eggs, liver, fish, especially sardines, green vegetables, prunes.
Calcium	Milk, cheese, fish, green vegetables, nuts, figs.
Iodine	Fish.

Note: Vitamins A & D are fat soluble. Vitamins C & B are water soluble. There is not sufficient scientific evidence to support the relevance of vitamin E to health in human beings.

enriched as it is with so many vitamin supplements, needs to give a thought to the daily intake of vitamins and minerals. Almost without exception, we are free of any vitamin deficiency. Unless we are prescribed vitamin supplements by a doctor, none are necessary to keep us in good health. Taking more vitamins than our bodies require does not improve our health one jot.

Emphasis is placed on vitamins and minerals because, while only eaten in minute traces, they are essential for healthy body metabolism. The word 'vitamin' itself means 'life-giving'.

Proteins

Proteins are of two sorts – first and second class. First-class proteins, sometimes described as 'complete', contain all the amino acids needed to repair damaged tissues and are usually animal proteins, e.g. meat, fish, cheese, eggs, milk and

Vitamins and minerals and the body processes for which they are essential

Vitamin	**Body process**
A	Health of skin, mucous membranes, eyes.
B_1	Health of brain, nerves, heart muscle.
B_2	Health of skin, hair, nails.
B_6	Essential in childhood and pregnancy.
Biotin	Health of skin and hair.
Niacin	Essential for normal growth.
B_3	Helps to protect against infection by building up antibodies.
Folic acid	Healthy blood cells.
B_{12}	Healthy blood cells.
C	Healthy mucous membranes, resistance to infections.
D	Regulates absorption, metabolism and excretion of calcium.
K	Essential for blood clotting, helps wound healing.

Mineral	
Iron	Health of red blood cells.
Calcium	Growth and health of bones and teeth.
Iodine	Needed for the healthy function of the thyroid gland.

dairy products. Second-class proteins, 'incomplete', do not contain as comprehensive a range of substances and are usually vegetable in origin, e.g. peas, beans, lentils, soya and the so-called pulses.

Proteins are crucial to our health because they provide eight of the twenty-two essential amino acids which the body must have in order to carry on its normal metabolism and growth. Although protein is essential for body growth we need surprisingly little pure protein each day – just about three and a half ounces, which you will get from a good helping of scrambled eggs, a thick slice of gammon, a fillet of fish or a joint of chicken.

Calories

Three different kinds of food provide our calories: carbohydrates, fats and proteins. Proteins and carbohydrates contain approximately the same number of calories per ounce – about 100 as a rule of thumb. Fats, however, contain twice as much, so if you want to reduce your calorie intake, the obvious way to do it is to cut back on fats. Fats, paradoxically, can sometimes help you to control your appetite in that they lie in your stomach for a long time and give you a sense of repletion.

What is a calorie and why are diets and dieticians so keen on them? In nutritional terms a calorie is a measurement of energy. So a food which contains many calories per ounce will give you more energy than one with a low calorific value. In strict scientific terms a calorie is a measurement of heat, and in dietetic terms heat is energy. Calories become important in dieting because if we do not use up all the energy we take in our food, the excess is deposited as fat. The only way we can know if we are taking in too many calories is by counting up the number of calories in the food we eat. If we are taking too many we must reduce the number of calories we eat per day to lose weight. You need to take in 3500 fewer calories than your body needs to lose a pound in weight. You lose it because your body burns up its own energy by getting its calories from your fat.

If we eat food that contains more calories than we need there is only one thing that can happen – we shall gain weight. It follows that there is only one way to get rid of fat and that is to take in fewer calories than we need. In doing so we force our bodies to make up the deficit by burning up our own fat. As we use up our own fat we lose weight. To keep our weight steady we must eat the amount of food, in terms of calories, that we need and no more.

The number of calories we need varies with sex (as a general rule men need more than women because, on average, they are more active), with the work we do (manual work requires more calories than sedentary work), with age (we need more calories at twenty-five than at sixty) and with the way we are made.

Calories required by men and women at varying ages

Age in years	Male	Female
5	1700	1700
15	2900	2300
25	2700–3600	2211–2700
45	2600–2900	2200–2500
60	2500	2000

There is no doubt that some people burn up food more efficiently than others. These are the fortunate people who can eat what they like and stay thin. The less fortunate have to be constantly careful about their diet. No one can change the rate at which their body metabolizes food and even though it seems that you are eating very little, possibly considerably less than your friends, if you are not losing weight you are still eating more than you need and you must cut back even further. Many people who are slim need, and naturally eat, very little. They very often have a limited appetite which acts as a brake and holds back their normal food intake to as little as a thousand calories a day without any effort whatsoever. Fat people on the other hand generally have hearty appetites that are not easily satiated and are more difficult to control. They seem to lack the 'I am full' reflex.

Obesity

Obesity is a fatal disease; it shortens your life by putting an extra burden on your heart, lungs, bones, joints and muscles. The obese have a greater tendency than normal to suffer from heart and chest complaints, joint and muscle disorders, arthritis and backache.

Obesity can be the main cause of adult diabetes. Diabetes is caused by a lack, or relative lack, of the hormone insulin which is necessary for the metabolism of carbohydrates; if you are overeating, and especially if you are overeating carbohydrates, the total body output of insulin is mopped up during the metabolism of excessive quantities of starchy food; insulin production cannot keep pace with demand and may eventually be exhausted; the body can no longer metabolize carbohydrates efficiently and the blood sugar rises – this is diabetes. This form, usually called adult-type diabetes, can often be rectified by the simple expedient of cutting down on starchy foods, thereby allowing the body's insulin supply to cope with the intake of carbohydrate, while simultaneously losing weight. One of the reasons why obesity can shorten life is that the complications of diabetes can be life-threatening. They include cataracts, kidney disease, high blood-pressure and heart disease.

Slimming

It is possible to burst a few balloons about slimming:

1 There is no substitute for will-power, self-control and perseverance.

2 You are fat because you eat too much.

3 Most people who are overweight require much less food than they think they need.

4 There is no known food which is slimming.

5 Being overweight is not due to the retention of fluid; healthy people do not retain fluid.

6 Thinking 'thin' does help some people to lose weight.

Despite all the diet sheets and dieting tricks, nibbler's diet, sweet-tooth's diet, film star's diet, crash diets, etc., the only way to lose weight is to take in fewer calories, that is to *eat less food*. If you are to do this, you must become a calorie counter and familiar with the calorie content of most of the foods you eat. Furthermore, you are going to have to weigh out all of the food you eat. Few people can lose weight unless they reduce their calorie intake to less than 1500 calories per day. Having been a failed dieter myself for something like twenty-five years, and having tried every tip in the book, here are my golden rules for what they are worth:

1 Obsessively record the calorific value of everything you eat during the day.

2 Try to restrict the calorie value of any meal to between 300–500 calories.

3 At six o'clock in the evening tot up all the calories you have eaten. Deduct the total from 1000. Whatever is left over is the number of calories you can take that night.

4 Don't take a calorie more.

On this regimen and others that are similar, many people have lost as much as three stones in nine months. To help you through that awful nine months here are a few suggestions which seem to help most slimmers:

1 Try to keep slimming uppermost in your mind. Keep a diary, read books, follow charts, talk to people and exchange notes with friends who are dieting.

2 Keep a good supply of low-calorie food in the house and in the fridge for those weak moments when you have to eat something – low calorie foods like fruit and raw vegetables, low-fat plain yoghurt, low-fat cottage cheese, etc.

3 Many people find they have quite a lot of will power if they can share their weight problem with other people, so find a friend or a group of dieters for support. Guilt is one of the best friends any slimmer can have.

4 Drink a glass of water just before a meal. It will take away the hunger pangs by adding volume to your stomach.

5 Stop taking sugar altogether, *now*. Best of all, learn to like unsweetened food but, if you must, start using artificial sweeteners for everything, especially cooking.

6 If your work means that you have to eat a lot of business lunches, work out a 500-calorie meal which you can have in any restaurant. My own favourite is a slice of melon or consommé to start, grilled fish or smoked salmon as a main course with a mixed salad and lemon juice dressing, then fresh fruit and black coffee.

7 One of the quickest ways to find out if you have put on any weight is to slip into your tightest pair of jeans at least once a week.

8 Don't throw dieting to the wind if you commit one misdemeanour. Try to think in a longer time scale – not just twenty-four hours ahead. Think of your body's needs in terms of a week. It is not difficult to compensate for that bar of chocolate by being careful over the next six days.

9 Always take the stairs instead of a lift or an escalator.

10 Eschew lemonade and sweet fizzy drinks. Always have a supply of low-calorie drinks in the house.

11 Remember most cravings last only a few minutes. If you can control it for that long you've beaten it.

12 Once you are down to your ideal weight save yourself the agony of having to diet regularly again by never allowing yourself to put on more than two or three pounds without taking corrective action.

Height and weight chart

Height (without shoes)	Women (2 lb. included for light indoor clothes)	Men (3 lb. included for light indoor clothes)
4 ft. 10 in.	7 st. 8 lb.	
4 11	7 11	
5 0	8 0	
5 1	8 3	9 st. 7 lb.
5 2	8 7	9 10
5 3	8 9	10 0
5 4	8 12	10 3
5 5	9 1	10 7
5 6	9 5	10 11
5 7	9 9	11 2
5 8	9 12	11 6
5 9	10 2	11 10
5 10	10 5	12 1
5 11	10 10	12 6
6 0		12 10
6 1		13 1
6 2		13 6
6 3		13 11

Having achieved your ideal weight you really must never return to the bad eating habits that made you overweight in the first place; you must believe that you have changed your eating pattern for life. If not, you risk becoming overweight again. These tables will give men in their forties some idea of when their weight becomes a danger:

Height	Weight (up to 45 years of age)	Weight (45–50 years of age)
5 ft. 6 in.	12 st. 8 lb.	12 st. 13 lb.
5 8	13 3	13 10
5 10	13 13	14 7
6 0	14 10	15 5

Danger weights for women are not available since women seldom suffer from coronary heart disease before they reach the menopause. However, it is worth remembering that anyone who is more than ten pounds overweight is putting a strain on their heart, and anyone who is more than a stone overweight should take drastic steps to reduce.

What we eat

Never before have people living in the developed world been exposed to such a varied and exciting diet. On the whole, however, this richness of choice has been abused. It has not led us to take advantage of hightly nutritious foods; on the contrary, the tendency has been to concentrate on producing refined and super-refined foods which bear hardly any relationship in consistency, appearance and taste to the raw materials from which they are made. Moreover, in the refining process much of the goodness may be lost.

Because we require that food be stored for long periods, many foods contain chemical additives to preserve them. Many others contain chemicals which 'improve' their flavour and enhance their colour. At present there are almost three thousand approved additives in use in the food industry. They have obvious advantages from which we all benefit, but occasionally research throws up information which shows some to be not quite as harmless as was first thought. During the war a bleach called agene was added to flour to whiten it; later research showed it to be toxic and it was withdrawn. Many colorants have come under a cloud over the past few years, usually because they are found to have harmful effects on animals, but the relevance of these findings to human beings is not known. Monosodium glutamate, a commonly used flavour-improver, is known to cause allergies in some sensitive people. Even saccharin has recently come under fire because it causes cancer in a particular species of rodent when given at many times the human dose over a long period of time. The health authorities are vigilant in watching out for public hazards and are quick to withdraw an additive which is shown to be in any way dangerous. Others are allowed to remain in use after a thorough investigation, e.g., nitrates used in the curing and colouring of bacon.

The purity of food may be tampered with even before it is processed. Very few crops which provide us with food are grown free of chemicals. Farmers and nutritionists alike find themselves in a cleft stick; without insecticides our crops can be damaged and without fertilizer they produce a poor yield. So entirely natural food is not necessarily the best food.

One-time favourite foods become discredited and some of the foods our mothers insisted on us eating have been relegated to a much lower status. Who can forget the spinach legend, built mainly on the foundation of Popeye's instant strength after gulping a tinful, which must have been responsible for many well-meaning parental exhortations to eat up; misplaced all of them. Spinach contains a chemical which, if eaten in large quantities, can deplete the body stores of bone-building calcium. Even more ironic, while it is an excellent source of iron, the same chemical not only prevents the absorption of the iron in spinach, but will prevent the absorption of iron from other foods eaten at the same meal. And so instead of being a supplier of iron, it drains iron from the body.

One of the major problems with refined foods is that essential roughage is removed along with minerals and vitamins during the refining process. To counteract this, calcium and iron are added to bread and vitamins A and D are added to margarine. Nevertheless what we are generally left with in super-refined food is a source of calories which provides no goodness, or very little.

Not all refined foods, however, are entirely without merit, nor are all so-called junk foods bad. Some of them can provide essential nutrients. A meal of hamburger, chips and a milkshake can give us a substantial share of our basic daily requirements of proteins, vitamins, minerals and calories in fairly well-balanced proportions. Beans, even though they come in a tin and in tomato sauce, are an excellent source of protein and calories. Fish-fingers are better than no fish at all.

While one would always wish to encourage good eating habits in children, you should never force a child to eat. To my mind it is better that children eat meat in the form of beefburgers and vegetables in the form of frozen beans, peas and sweetcorn, than that they should not eat any of these foods at all. Milk is an excellent food and should be taken by all children, but it does not have to be taken in the form of plain milk. It can just as well be ice-cream, custard or a flavoured drink. A good rule is to have some fresh fruit every day, but it can be whatever kind your child likes – a fresh tomato is better than most, if that is his predilection. The roughage in his diet can be augmented by cereals at breakfast, and wholemeal bread – which once exposed to, most children prefer to over-refined ready-sliced white, especially if you bake it yourself!

For the past few years we have been going through a swing back to natural, uncontaminated 'health' foods, and in general this can only be a good trend. More and more people are eating fresh foods as opposed to cooked foods. Fresh vegetables are much better for us than cooked vegetables because most cooking processes destroy the vitamin C content. Vegetables should never be cooked for more than a few minutes if you want to preserve the vitamin C. The return to wholewheat, rough-ground flour is an excellent move. This is because it is a source of roughage in our diet, a constituent which has become almost non-existent in the diet of most people in the western world. The number of people who eschew soft, white, pulpy, non-bulky sliced bread in favour of the much more wholesome wholewheat bread is rightly growing. Dried fruits and nuts contain many calories but are always preferable to sweets and chocolates. Stewed prunes, apricots and figs will not only provide a pleasant snack and useful roughage but will do much to alleviate constipation, without recourse to a patent medicine.

The fad for natural vitamins, which is encouraged by health-food shops, is to be deprecated. 'Natural' vitamins are a confidence trick – they are no different nutritionally from synthetic vitamins, they just cost you more. In any case, very few vitamin preparations are made solely from natural sources. To guarantee their effectiveness most manufacturers have found it necessary to mix vitamins from natural and synthetic sources.

'Natural' foods, i.e. those which are grown without the aid of synthetic additives, are not necessarily any healthier than other foods, particularly those with a high fat content like nuts, eggs, cheese, milk and avocado pears. Sea salt and soya sauce, by the way, are no better for you than ordinary table salt.

Diet and disease

In some cases, what people eat can be responsible for their ill-health. Doctors have found that foods can be related to colitis, migraine, allergies and constipation. With the exception of constipation, the association between the food and the medical condition is nearly always due to an allergy.

Allergy to food can take various forms, and in the medical records one can find reports of allergies to almost all foods. By far the commonest are: nuts; fruits, such as strawberries and raspberries; tinned meats, such as tongue; a wide variety of fish, particularly shell-fish; and drinks such as cocoa and tea. The allergy may cause very little discomfort, like nettle-rash which disappears in a few minutes, or it may cause a severe reaction throughout the whole body in which case the face, lips and the eyes become very swollen and itchy. The reaction may involve the stomach and the intestine with abdominal pain and diarrhoea and, in some people, can give cause for concern. With medical treatment, however, the patient can be well again in a few days. The most serious form is a long-term debilitating condition of the bowel called ulcerative colitis which is thought by some physicians to be an allergy to milk, possibly even to toothpaste.

Malabsorption syndrome is also very serious, particularly when it occurs in children, and it is usually due to an allergy to gluten which is a protein in cereals. The allergy causes malabsorption of many foodstuffs because of the allergic inflammation in the lining of the intestine. The only way to remain free of this condition is to eat a gluten-free diet.

Migraine sufferers report that an attack may be precipitated by eating chocolate, cheese, any rich or fatty food or by drinking a glass of sherry. Allergy to food may play a part in the cause of migraine, but there are many other factors, such as stress, lack of sleep, or excitement, which are just as important.

Constipation is a combination of many factors. First, there is the human obsession with bowel habit and the misconception that one needs to empty the bowels daily. This is quite wrong: bowel evacuation every three or four days is perfectly normal and opening need not be induced artificially. Then there is the neglect to heed the call to stool because you are too busy. If we ignore the call to stool for long enough the bowel becomes lazy and does not bother to give us the message. Most people then start to take purgatives which make the bowel even lazier. The only way to break this circle is to recultivate good habits. But probably the most important factor is correcting your diet: a diet of soft pulpy foods with a low residue gives the bowel very little to work on and produces very little stool, but the addition of roughage will correct this. You can take roughage naturally in fruit, vegetables and cereal, and adding bran to your breakfast cereal is a good habit to cultivate.

The food we eat can change the way our bodies handle drugs. At its simplest this means that if you take a drug on a full stomach it will be longer before you feel the effect of the drug because the presence of food in the stomach slows down its absorption. If you have diarrhoea, food is hurrying through the intestine and that may also interfere with the absorption of a drug, and therefore you may be deprived of its benefit. This is important for women taking the oral contraceptive pill who have an attack of diarrhoea: the pill may not be absorbed and its contraceptive efficacy can be interrupted. At such a time extra precautions should be taken.

There is a group of drugs used for the treatment of depression called mono-amine oxidase inhibitors which react with certain foods and increase the blood-pressure. The foods to avoid if you take mono-amine oxidase drugs are matured cheeses, protein extract, such as Marmite or Bovril, alcoholic drinks, red wine and in particular Chianti, broad-bean pods and protein foods that are not fresh when eaten, for instance those which have been 'hung'.

There is no doubt that the food we eat is connected with tooth decay. We all know that sweets and sweet drinks encourage the development of 'caries'. Sweet substances are bad for the teeth because they lead to the formation of plaque or tartar, a soft, creamy deposit on the teeth which becomes hard and chalky. It collects in the spaces between our teeth and gradually erodes, undermines and finally destroys the gum margins by the formation of pockets in which bacteria flourish. Because of hard-hitting propaganda about dental care and hygiene, the final stage, pyorrhoea, is now rare.

While correct brushing of the teeth, regular use of dental floss and frequent visits to the dentist can do much to ensure the health of your teeth, research done at the Royal Dental Hospital in London has shown that there are culprits other than sweet starchy foods that cause tooth decay. Cheese, for instance, is particularly prone to cause plaque. The apple or raw carrot which as children we were encouraged to chew on last thing at night 'to clean your teeth' are no more cariogenic than some other foods, but they do not *clean* the teeth as was thought, nor do they protect them from decay.

Unless we take special steps to see that it does not happen, most of us suffer from a shortage of fibre in our diet. Fibre or roughage can only be found in fruit, vegetables and cereals. Recent research has compared the amount of roughage in the diet of African tribesmen and in people from developed countries and then examined the different patterns of diseases suffered by these two groups. The startling results showed that the Africans, with fibre-rich diets, had a very low incidence of many common western diseases. The results have been extrapolated to the conclusion that it is necessary to increase the amount of fibre in our diet. Although the mechanism is not known, doctors believe that the presence of fibre in the diet diminishes the tendency to develop such commonplace conditions as appendicitis, diverticulitis, colitis, bowel cancer, thrombosis, heart disease, piles and varicose veins. One of the reasons why it is thought that fibre can protect us from these illnesses is that it retains water in the bowel. Concomitant with the retention of water, it retains harmful substances which might otherwise be absorbed into the blood-stream. Our daily fibre requirement can be fulfilled by the simple expedient of adding two tablespoons of bran to our diet each day.

Research over the last ten or fifteen years has shown that our diets contain what might be called 'risk' foods. These foods are associated, amid controversy, with the development of fatal diseases of the heart. While the dispute rages, most doctors would advocate that the intake of these foods, wherever possible, should be reduced, and in some instances eliminated altogether from the diet. Risk foods would be:

1 Foods which contain large amounts of saturated (or animal) fats.
2 Saturated (or animal) fats *per se*.
3 Foods which contain large amounts of cholesterol, e.g. egg yolk.
4 Foods which contain refined sugar.

For a detailed discussion of the effect of diet on heart disease see Chapter 4.

3 The Importance of Exercise

There are three main reasons why exercise is important to you: firstly, you will get more out of life; secondly, you will keep your body in good working order; and thirdly, you will protect yourself against many disabling diseases and a few fatal ones.

We all know grandmothers who have more energy than we have, seventy-year-olds who are still doing an hour's jogging every morning, middle-aged men and women who are as lithe and slender as they were in their teens – they are all having a whale of a time, a much better time than those of us who are a good deal younger but who are unfit and overweight. The fact cannot be ignored that people who are healthy and fit seem to enjoy everything more than those who are not. Not just because they have a different attitude to life, which they do, but because they have the physical and emotional capacity to get the most out of it. To get more out of life you need strength and vitality and vigour, and you will be better able to retain these qualities if you exercise regularly and stay fit.

What happens to our bodies when we exercise

Our bodies are machines with many working, interlocking, interdependent parts, and just like machines they become inefficient, develop weaknesses and faults and eventually seize up if left to lie idle. Like any machine, our bodies must be kept well maintained. They are designed to be exercised frequently and pushed to the limits of physical endurance. Only athletes seem to go in for the latter, but if we want to keep any degree of physical fitness it is necessary to put our muscles and joints through their paces, and exercise them to the point of fatigue. Only then will we be fit enough to cope with the urgent extra effort that is sometimes demanded of us.

A routine programme of exercise has more than an immediate pay-off because you are buying good health for possibly an additional decade at the end of your life. We do not have any proof that physical fitness automatically increases longevity, but we do know that unfit people are throwing away their chance to live a long and happy life because they are more likely to develop chest trouble, low back pain and arthritis. They also have a greater tendency to have accidents. More importantly, evidence is accumulating that people who do not exercise are more likely to have high blood-pressure and heart disease.

Let us take a look at what happens to our bodies when we exercise fairly strenuously – that means exercising large muscle groups like the muscles of the thighs, legs, arms and shoulders. When muscles are exercised they do continuous work. This work involves regular and frequent contraction and relaxation of the muscle over a period of time, say fifteen to thirty minutes. When a muscle contracts and relaxes it uses up energy and oxygen. Energy is stored in the muscle in the form of sugar. Energy is also transported to the muscle via the blood in the form of blood sugar. The supply of oxygen to the muscle is dependent on an efficient and plentiful blood-supply.

If a muscle goes on contracting and relaxing for any length of time, the stores of sugar eventually become depleted. If exercise continues, sugar cannot be replaced fast enough from sugar in the blood. Skeletal muscle has a special property which allows it to go on exercising even though its source of energy has been exhausted. It builds up an energy debt, but it can only keep going for a time, dependent on the amount and difficulty of the work demanded of the muscle, after this energy debt has begun to accumulate, until a severe pain ensues. When the muscle stops exercising it rebuilds its energy stores and pays off the debt; subsequently it builds up a credit balance of sugar stores.

When a muscle is exercising its consumption of oxygen may double, triple or even quadruple. As the only source of oxygen to the muscle is via the bloodstream, the increased need for oxygen means that the blood has to be pumped to the muscle twice, three times or even four times as fast as when the muscle is resting. The only way that this can be accomplished is for the heart to work harder and pump blood to the muscle faster. The heart responds by beating faster and the pulse rate rises. Not only that, but with each beat, the muscles of the heart contract more strongly and push out a greater volume of blood. This increased work-load of the heart is reflected in the lungs, because it is essential that the increased volume of blood is well oxygenated. It is therefore very important that oxygenation of the blood is efficient.

The blood is oxygenated in the lungs. With each intake of breath, we fill the millions of air spaces in the lungs with air. Blood which is circulating around these air sacs soaks up as much oxygen as possible and transports it to the muscles that are working where it releases it. Because of this increased 'hunger' for oxygen on the part of exercising muscles, we breathe more deeply to get more air into the lungs and breathe faster to improve oxygenation of the blood.

As we become fitter, the heart is able to cope more easily with this extra work. The pulse rate does not increase as much as it did previously because the fitter heart muscle is able to beat more strongly and push out a larger volume of blood per beat. When the heart muscle was less strong it was able to increase the volume only by increasing the number of beats per minute. Similarly our lungs become more efficient. We are able to expand our lungs to a greater volume than before thereby increasing the efficiency of oxygenation without having to rely on increasing the number of breaths per minute. Furthermore, as our muscles become more accustomed to exercise they are able to go on exercising for longer without building up a sugar debt. All these improvements represent the achievement of fitness.

Here are some guidelines about exercising:

1 We should do the right kind of exercises to improve our fitness.

2 We should gradually increase the length and strength of exercises to achieve the level of fitness suitable for our age.

3 We should exercise regularly to maintain that level of fitness.

A simple exercise programme

Al Murray, national and olympic coaching adviser and director of the City Gym in London, believes that any exercise programme must contain three sorts of exercise. He defines the exercises as: *mobility exercises*; *strengthening exercises*; *heart and lung exercises*.

Mobility exercises are designed to move all the major muscles and joints through their complete range of movement. When you have achieved mobility fitness you will be able to move, stretch, twist and turn in all directions with freedom.

Al's strengthening exercises are designed to enable our bodies to cope with the extra effort we are sometimes called upon to make in special circumstances. So we build in a safety margin or extra strength over and above normal requirements. It is important that we do have this reserve because when it is not there, making a sudden and extreme effort can result in damaged muscles, ligaments and tendons, and even a slipped disc. To build up those extra resources you have to increase the duration and force of the exercise you take, a little at a time.

The heart and lungs are only exercised when we increase our oxygen requirements above normal. As described, this happens when the exercise involves large muscle groups. Every exercise which does this is suitable to keep the heart and lungs in good shape. Such suitable exercise would be running, jogging, swimming, cycling, rowing.

Before you can aim for the level of fitness for your age you must know how *unfit* you are. This can be assessed in a simple way by examining the response of your heart to strenuous exercise – strenuous exercise being that which increases the oxygen requirements of the body above normal. You measure this by taking your pulse. An unfit heart will start to beat very fast when you exercise strenuously, because it is the only way that it can pump more blood around the body to keep up with the demand for oxygen. A fit heart, however, will not beat as fast because it can pump out more blood with each beat than an unfit heart. It goes without saying that anyone who has any heart trouble at all, or who has been told by their doctor that they have had heart trouble, should not undertake any of the heart and lung exercises. If you are in doubt you should consult your doctor first.

To perform a simple test to see how fit you are, run on the spot for a short time, say thirty seconds, and then take your pulse. If you are fit your pulse rate will be at your personal pulse rating; if you are unfit it will be above it; if you are extremely fit it will be below it. To calculate your personal pulse rate you do the following:

1 Subtract your age from 200.
2 Subtract a handicap of 40 for not being fit.
3 The figure that results is your *personal pulse rate.*

If you are forty-two years of age, you will subtract that figure from 200, which leaves 158, take away 40, leaving 118, and that is your personal pulse rating.

How to take your pulse

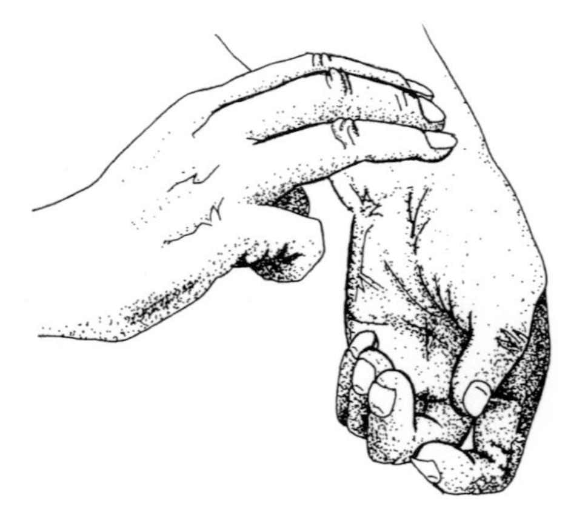

You take your pulse by placing the tips of the three fingers of your right hand down the thumb edge of the undersurface of your left wrist with the palm of the left hand facing upwards. If your fingers are in the correct position, you will feel the radial artery throbbing underneath your fingers with each beat of the heart. To get an accurate timing of your pulse you should count the number of beats for fifteen seconds, and then multiply by four to get the rate per minute.

The aim of heart and lung exercises is to maintain this pulse rate for a period of ten minutes of continuous exercising. As a margin of safety the pulse must go no higher than the one you have calculated. If, after running on the spot for thirty seconds, your pulse rate is at your personal rating then you can continue and you should keep on taking your pulse every minute or so. If, after thirty seconds, your pulse rate is higher than your personal rating, you must wait and rest until your pulse comes down. You should continue to do this every half minute or so if the exercise increases your pulse rate beyond your personal rating. When you are very unfit you will have to stop and start your exercises frequently for rest periods, but it is very important to do so to make certain that your heart is not under strain.

As you improve your fitness you will be able to go for longer periods without raising your pulse rate above your personal rating and you will have to rest less often. You will have achieved your goal when you are able to exercise continuously for ten minutes without your pulse rate going above your personal rating. To do these exercises properly you are going to have to become very familiar with taking your own pulse.

Al Murray's well-proven schedule of mobility exercises include: arm circling, side bends, trunk, knee and hip bends; trunk, head and arm rotating; and alternate ankle reaching. Al recommends that these exercises should be done at a relaxed even tempo. Progress is achieved by gradually increasing the range of movement. There is no need to increase the speed of the exercises or the number of the repetitions above ten or twelve. Breathing should be kept free and easy to fit the rhythm of the movements.

Good strengthening exercises, all in slightly different forms from easy to difficult, include: press-ups for the arms and shoulders; straight leg raising for the abdominal muscles; and leg exercising involving knee bends. You should start by doing all of these exercises in their easiest form and only progress to the more difficult forms when you can complete the schedule without discomfort.

The aim of strengthening exercises as you would expect is to increase the strength of the muscles. One should never be in a hurry to rush these exercises beyond your personal pulse rating. You should wait until you can do the full number of repetitions without raising your personal pulse rate before you increase to a higher number of repetitions. So you should start with eight or ten repetitions of each. As you become stronger you should gradually increase the number to say twenty or thirty. When you can do the first eight repetitions comfortably you should progress to the next form of the exercise and again start from the lowest level and work up to twenty or thirty.

The heart and lung exercises should conform to the criteria I have already described and should include such exercises as: running on the spot; stepping on and off a bench (the bench should be no higher than eighteen inches); outdoor exercises such as running, jogging, cycling or swimming. After you have done an outdoor exercise for periods of ten continuous minutes for eight to ten weeks, you can try to raise your pulse rate in steps of no more than five, to a maximum of twenty. Very gradually you can also try to increase the duration of your exercise.

Once you have achieved your level of fitness the maintenance of this fitness can take up very little of your time and effort. In a book entitled *F/40 Fitness on Forty Minutes a Week*, Dr Michael Carruthers and Al Murray show how you can do just that. The exercise sessions need not be more frequent than three times a week and none of them need last more than fifteen or twenty minutes. Each exercise session should include the mobility exercises already discussed. And these do not progress either in terms of number of repetitions or the speed at which you do them. You should include the strengthening exercises, gradually progressing through the stage of difficulty and upwards from eight to ten repetitions to twenty or thirty. The heart and lung exercises should also be carried out and should always be monitored by taking your pulse. You can progress through a series of exercises such as the following regimens, always beginning each session with mobility exercises to loosen up:

1 Press-ups against a wall.
  Thigh-raising seated on a chair.
  Squats behind a chair back.

2 Press-ups on a table top.
  Straight leg-raising on a chair.
  Squats without a chair.
  Running on the spot.

3 Press-ups on a chair seat.
  Sit-ups from lying on the floor.
  Jumps from squatting position.
  Bench stepping.

4 Full press-ups on the floor.
  V-sits with heels on a chair.
  Star jumps.
  Jogging, cycling or swimming.

The motto of all exercise programmes is: take as much time as you need, work at your own rate and don't be in a hurry to progress fast.

Mobility exercises

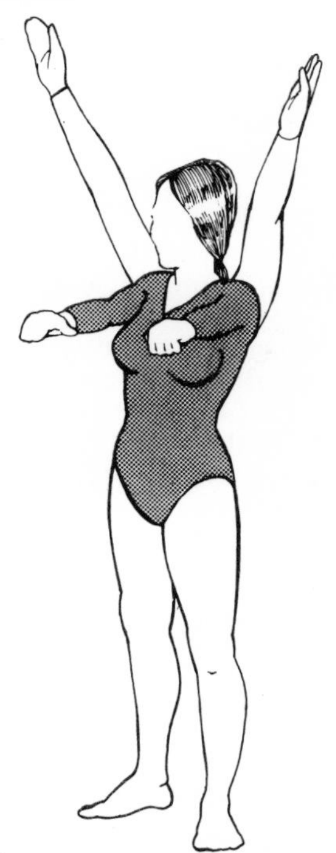

1 Arm circling.

Stand with your feet wide apart and your arms hanging loosely by your sides. Raise both arms forwards, upwards, backwards and sideways, in a circular motion, brushing your ears with your arms as you go past.

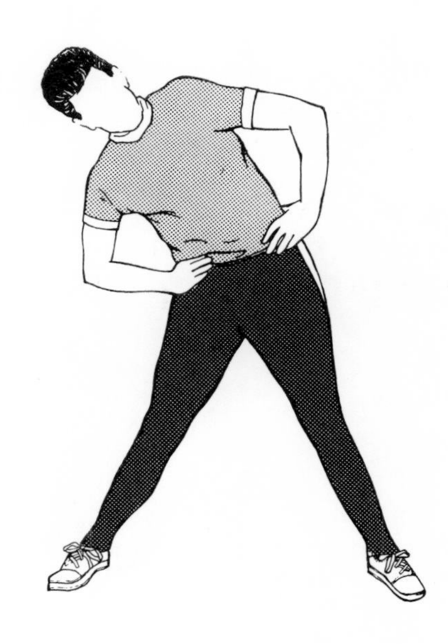

2 Side bends.

Stand with your feet wide apart and hands on hips. Bend first to the left and then to the right, keeping the head at right angles to the trunk.

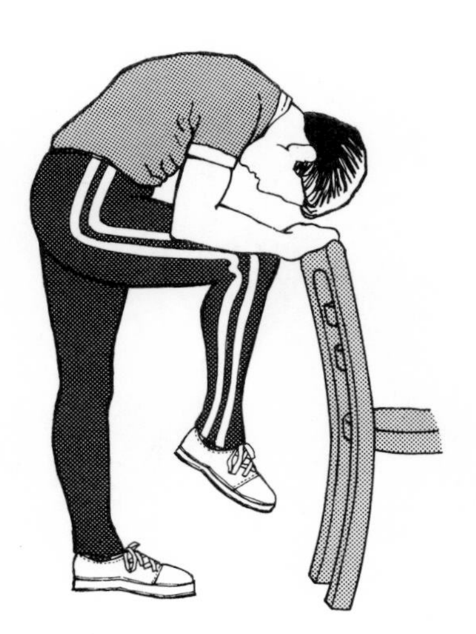

3 Trunk, knee and hip bends.

Stand 18 inches behind the back of a chair with your hands resting lightly on the back. Raise the left knee and bring the forehead down to meet it. Repeat with the right knee. This should be a long, strong movement so do not rush it. Once you are used to this exercise you can work from a standing position, without a chair.

Mobility exercises cont.

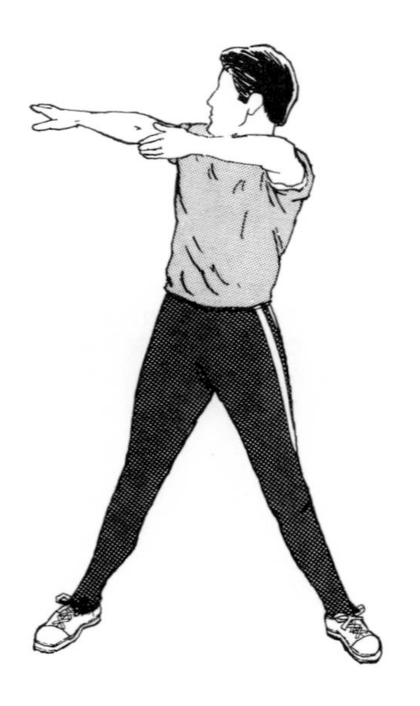

4 Head, arms and trunk rotating.

Stand with your feet wide apart, with hands and arms outstretched in front of your shoulders. Turn the head, arms and shoulder around to the left as far as you can go, bending the right arm across the chest, then repeat the movement to the right. Keep your hips and legs still throughout the exercise.

5 Alternate ankle reaching.

Stand with your feet wide apart, with both palms resting against the front of the upper left thigh. Relax the trunk forward as you slide both hands down the leg towards the left ankle. Return to starting position and repeat on the right. (N.B. Anyone suffering from back trouble should not pass the knees with the hands).

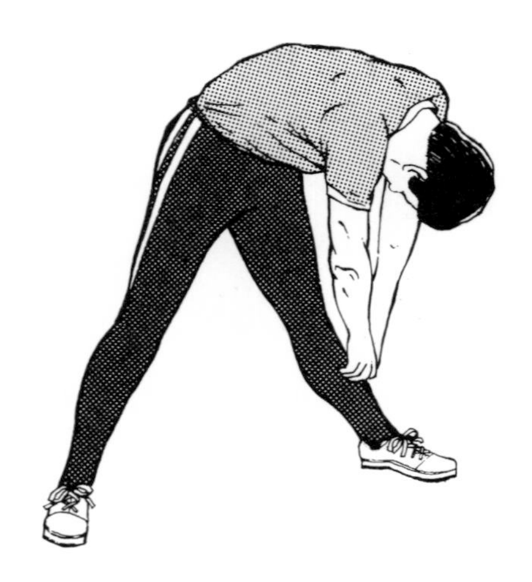

Stage one

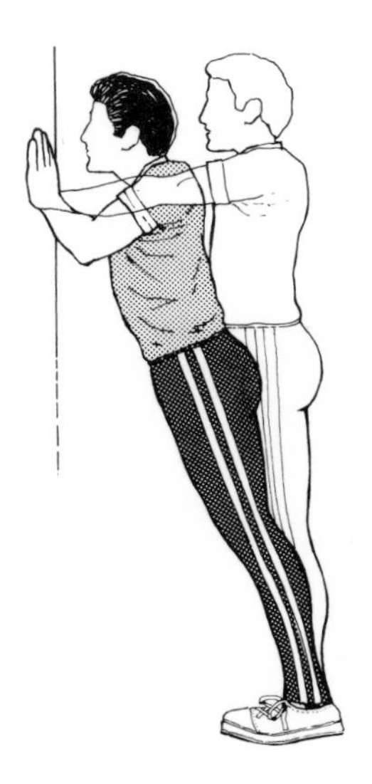

1 Press-ups against a wall.

Stand with hands on the wall 12 ins apart at shoulder height and arms straight. Stand on your toes, then bend the arms until the chest and chin touch the wall. Return to starting position by straightening arms.

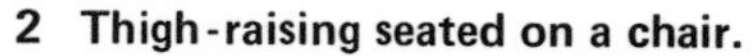

2 Thigh-raising seated on a chair.

Sit on the front part of the chair, legs straight and heels on the floor. Lean back and grip the sides of the seat for support. Bend the knees and bring the fronts of the thighs up to squeeze gently against the body.

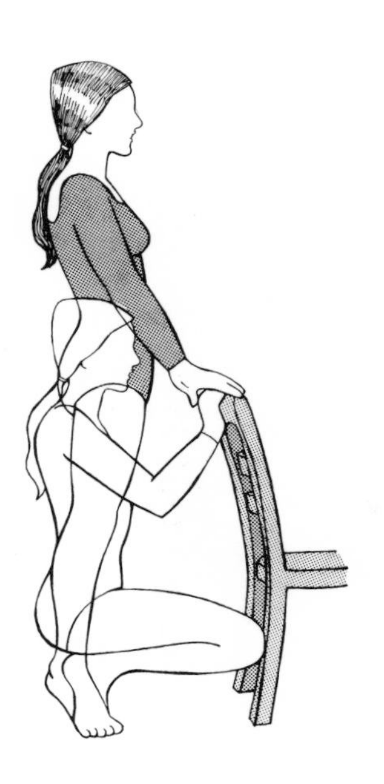

3 Squats holding a chair back.

Stand 18 ins behind a chair with your hands on the back. Lower the body into a squat, keeping the feet flat on the floor (women may stand on their toes at this point). Straighten both legs and come up on the toes, then return to squat position.

Stage two

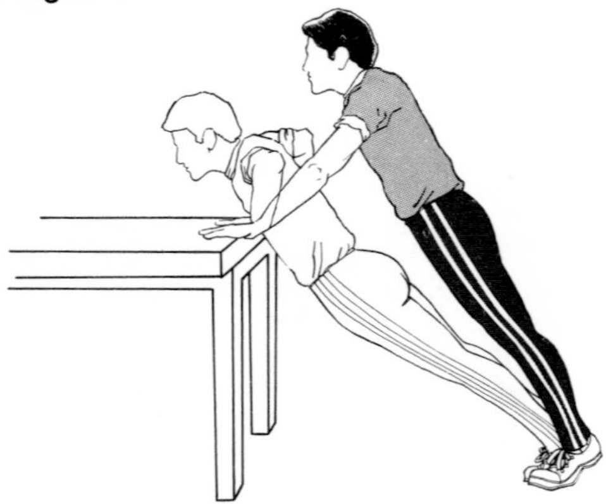

1 Press-ups on a table top.
Place hands 10 to 12 ins apart on a table (make sure it is safe). Bend arms keeping body straight until chest touches table, then return to starting position.

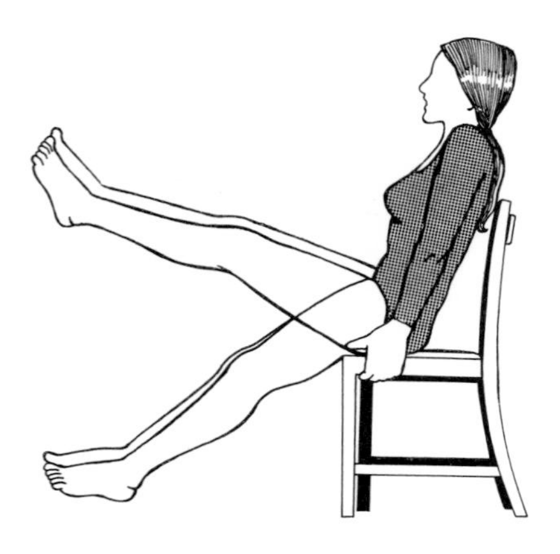

2 Straight leg-raising on a chair.
Sit on the front part of the chair with legs straight and heels on the floor. Lean back and grip sides of the seat for support. Keeping the legs straight, raise them as high as you can, then return to starting position.

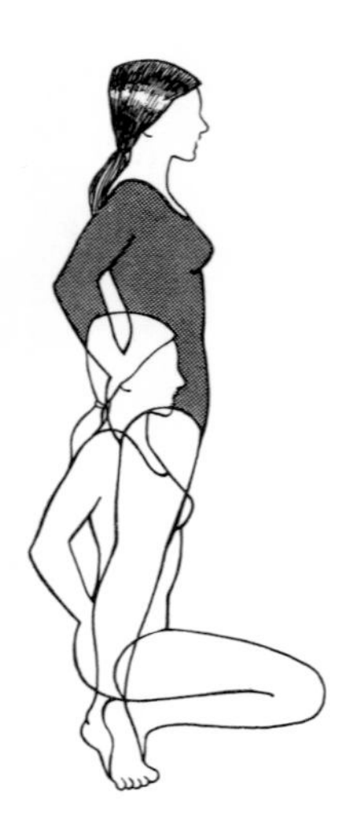

3 Squats without a chair.
Stand with feet slightly apart and hands on your hips. Lower the body into a squat, then straighten both legs and come up on the toes. Return to starting position.

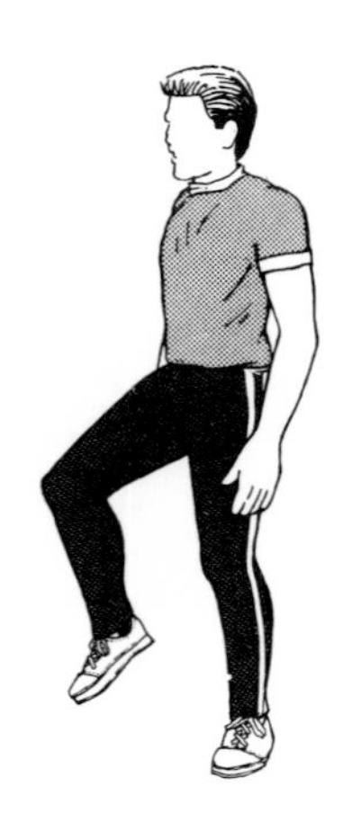

4 Running on the spot.
Stand with arms loosely by your sides and gently run on the spot. Do not begin by raising the knees high but aim to get them higher as you become fitter.

Stage three

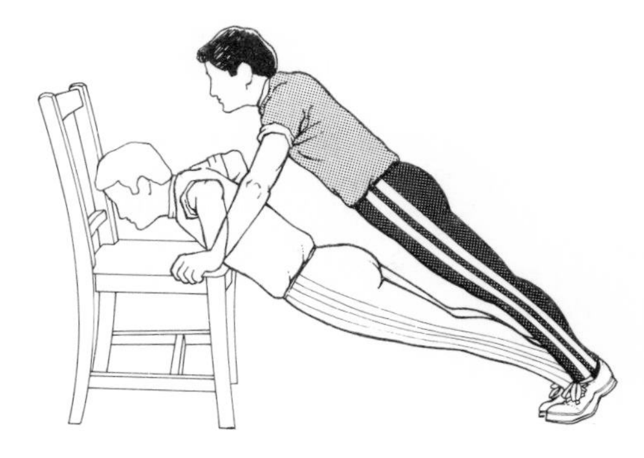

1 Press-ups on a chair seat.

Grip the sides of a chair seat. Bend your arms, keeping the body straight, until the chest touches the chair and then return to starting position. Be sure the chair is steady and that your head clears the back as you go down.

2 Sit-ups from lying on the floor.

Lie on your back with your legs slightly bent and your feet tucked under a heavy chair or couch. Arms should be stretched backwards. Swing up to sitting position, no further than where your hands can touch your ankles.

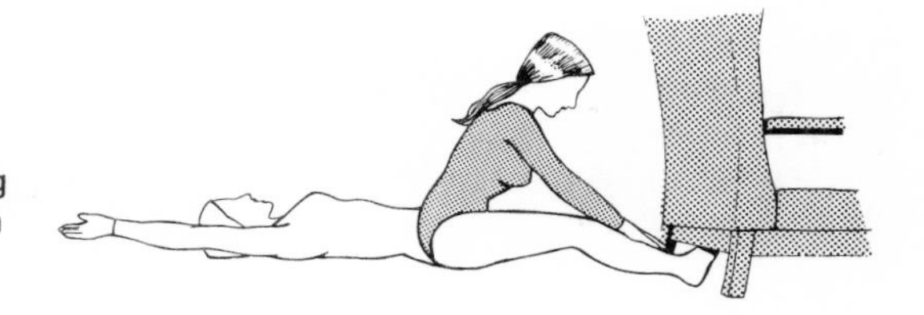

3 Jumps from squatting position.

Stand with feet slightly apart and hands on your hips. Lower the body into a squat, then come up fast so that your feet actually leave the floor, at first only a few inches, then a bit higher.

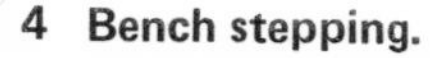

4 Bench stepping.

Take a low box or stool and stand 12 ins away from it with hands on hips. Step on to it first with right foot leading, then with left. Gradually increase height of bench to a maximum of 18 ins.

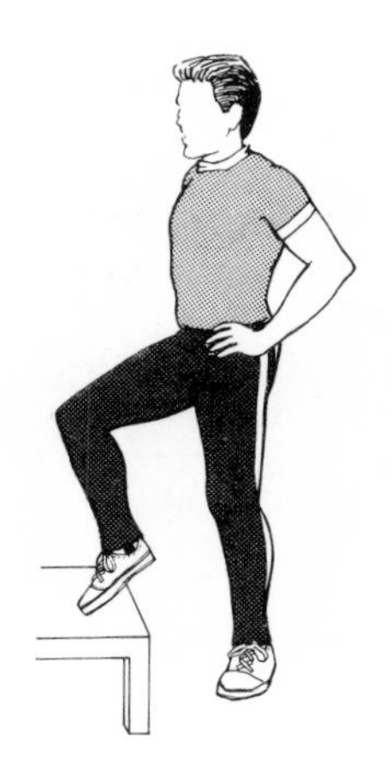

Stage four

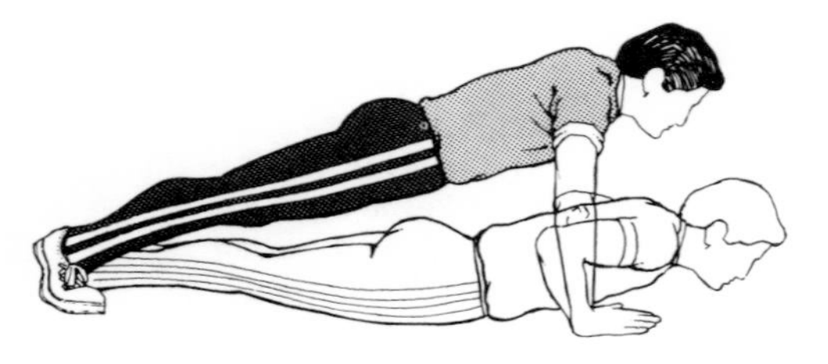

1 Full press-ups on the floor.

Place your hands on the floor directly under your shoulders with the fingers pointing forward. Chest and shoulders should be lowered slowly to touch the floor and then raised until the arms are straight. The back and legs should remain straight throughout.

2 V-sits with heels on a chair.

Lie on your back with your hands behind your head and your heels on the edge of a chair. Swing up to sitting position, allowing your knees to bend slightly as you do so.

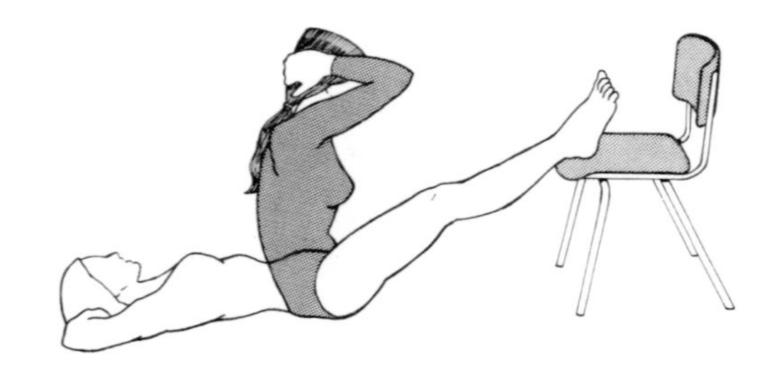

3 Star jumps.

Stand with feet a few inches apart, knees half bent and hands by the sides of your knees. Leap upwards into a star jump. As you land, bend the knees to take up the shock.

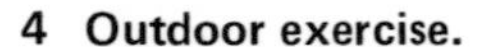

4 Outdoor exercise.

Choose between jogging, swimming or cycling and aim to do ten minutes continuously. You can improve fitness by increasing the duration of the exercise.

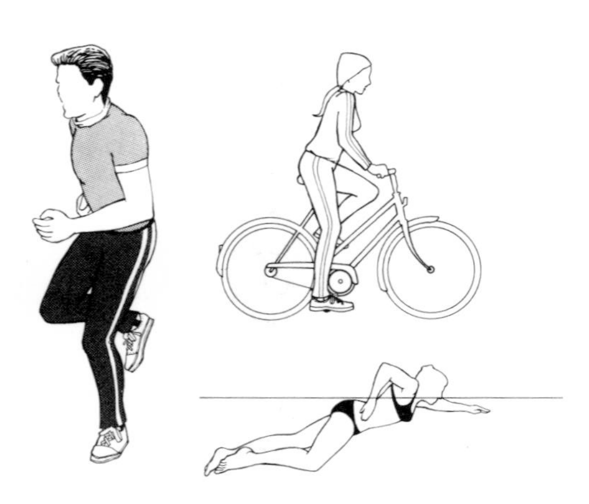

How to Keep a Healthy Heart

Keeping a healthy heart depends on four main factors – diet, exercise, avoidance of smoking and avoidance of too much stress. The tendency to have heart disease can be determined even before you are born; heart disease runs in families; it is more common in children of diabetics; and there is a higher incidence in the children of people who have high blood cholesterol levels.

Diet

The predisposition to develop heart disease in those of us who do not fall into any of these groups may, nonetheless, be determined in the cradle. The old idea of a beautiful bouncing baby was one that was fat and overweight. Investigation of fat metabolism in infants has shown that fat babies are likely to turn into fat adults. If you overfeed your baby you are encouraging bad habits for later life. It has been shown that the fat cells in fat babies can hold more fat than fat cells in babies of the proper weight, and that when fat babies grow up they have more fat cells than do normal babies. By encouraging your baby to eat too much you may be lighting the fuse which finally explodes as a heart attack in middle age.

The lay-public is under the impression that medical theories regarding the connection of some foods with heart disease come and go like fashions in clothes. This is not so, though all the theories have their believers and non-believers. The truth is probably a combination of them all so I would not hazard excluding any.

There is a statistical association between diets rich in saturated fats and coronary heart disease; this means that the more saturated fats you eat the more likely you are to die of a heart attack. The coronary arteries supply blood to the heart muscle to keep it pumping. In coronary artery disease, the arteries become narrowed due to deposits of fatty substances within their walls – like water pipes becoming furred up. People who die of heart attacks almost invariably have furred-up coronary arteries. In Europe, the Scandinavians, who eat most animal fat, suffer most heart attacks, while the Italians, who eat the least animal fat although a lot of vegetable fat, suffer least from heart attacks. In certain primitive tribes whose diet is mainly maize and beans with very little meat or eggs, heart disease is virtually unknown (see also p. 41).

Almost all animal fats are saturated and almost all vegetable fats are unsaturated. Saturated fats are 'saturated' with hydrogen atoms and this confers on them a high melting point; that is, they are solid at room temperature – lard, for instance. Unsaturated fats have empty spaces in their molecules instead of hydrogen atoms and this lowers their melting points; thus, they are liquid at room temperature, for instance, vegetable oil. It is thought that very unsaturated fat (polyunsaturated) may even *remove* some of the fatty deposits from the coronary arteries.

A good rule is to keep the amount of animal fat in your diet low, i.e. no more than one ounce per day, and to substitute vegetable oil for lard and soft margarine for butter whenever you can.

Foods vary in the amount of saturated and unsaturated fat they contain (the calorific values of saturated and unsaturated fats are identical).

Food	saturated fat %	unsaturated fat %	polyunsaturated fat %
Milk, butter, cheese	62	30	3
Beef	48	44	3
Margarine (Stork)	41	54	5
Margarine (Stork SB)	26	59	15
Chicken	32	37	26
Lamb	54	37	4
Liver	34	27	34
Herring	19	10	66
Olive oil	11	74	10
Corn oil	17.5	29	56.5
Sunflower oil	12	20	68

(Source: *The Sunday Times Book of Body Maintenance*, Michael Joseph)

We do not know exactly how cholesterol causes heart disease but a statistical association between the two has been proven. It is therefore wise to avoid foods which contain large quantities of cholesterol. The body can make good use of cholesterol: it is the starting substance for all the sex hormones, cortisol and related hormones, those that actually keep us alive. The yolk of eggs and salmon are particularly rich in cholesterol so as a preventative measure you should eat these foods sparingly and avoid them altogether if you have heart trouble.

Some research which was undertaken nearly forty years ago shows that the incidence of heart disease varies between districts where the drinking water is either hard or soft. It was shown unequivocally that the incidence of heart disease was lower in areas where the drinking water was harder. So if you are going to install a water softener in your domestic water supply, make sure that it leaves the drinking water untouched.

A fairly new hypothesis puts forward the view that the amount of roughage in the diet can affect the tendency to have heart disease (see p. 52). The exact mechanism by which fibre in the diet protects the heart from disease is not known but it is suggested that if your diet is low on roughage and high on low-bulk processed foods then your tendency to develop heart disease is increased. It follows that you should take active steps to make sure that your diet contains a fair amount of roughage in the form of cereals, vegetables and fibre supplements if necessary.

Here are a few dietary guidelines from the Royal College of Physicians on how to promote a healthy heart. Though you may have to change your lifestyle to follow them, you may well live longer as a result.

1 Reduce the fat in your diet. Replace most of the animal fat with unsaturated vegetable fat such as soft margarine, corn oil, soya bean oil or sunflower oil. Do not have more than half an ounce of butter a day. Never use lard or hard margarine for cooking.

2 Eat lean meat, e.g. beef, rather than fatty meat such as pork. Always cut the fat off meat if possible.

3 Try to eat less red meat and more white meat such as poultry and fish.

4 Grill food whenever you can, never fry it.

5 Make sure that you eat some fruit, or some green or root vegetables, to provide roughage, and if you cannot, take two tablespoons of fibre supplement or bran every day.

6 Do not eat more than one egg per day and try not to eat more than three eggs per week.

7 Avoid double cream whenever you can; take single rather than double cream if there is a choice.

The Royal College of Physicians recommends a very strict diet for people who suffer from heart disease, the aim being to reverse the condition which already exists. It recommends that meat is restricted to eight ounces a week, that soft margarines, high in polyunsaturated fats, are always used, that milk must always be skimmed, that no more than three eggs a week are eaten and that cheese be kept to a minimum, with cottage cheese used as a substitute. The intake of cakes, pastry and biscuits should be restricted. In fact, a vegetarian diet seems to be particularly suitable for people who have suffered from heart disease and, as already mentioned, certain communities who have a diet that is mainly vegetarian and contains very few dairy products have a reduced incidence of heart disease.

Exercise

Everyone should exercise regularly. Even middle-aged people who have not exercised on any regular basis for years can start immediately, as long as they begin gradually. Only people who have been told that they have some form of heart disease, or people who are very overweight, should consult their doctors before starting on an exercise programme. If you develop any distressing symptoms during exercise, however, you should consult your doctor.

Exercise keeps the heart and muscles in good trim as described in Chapter 3 and has the additional benefit of reducing the blood cholesterol. It has been shown that exercise speeds up the metabolism which has a cholesterol-lowering effect on the blood. This effect can be increased if you exercise about forty-five minutes after food when the metabolism is already slightly raised by the recent meal. So if you exercise regularly and frequently you will be helping to normalize your blood cholesterol and possibly to ward off the deposition of fat in the walls of your arteries which is often the forerunner of heart disease.

Regular and frequent exercise can also protect you from having a heart attack even if one of the major blood-vessels to the heart becomes blocked. This is because strenuous exercise opens up a network of small interlacing blood-vessels which provide a subsidiary blood-supply to the heart muscle. If we are inactive for any length of time this network tends to close down, like unused paths which become overgrown. The anastomoses, as they are called, are always present to be opened up again however, and as you gradually increase the strength and frequency of your exercises the anastomoses become patent. The anastomotic arteries provide an alternative path for blood to reach any section of heart muscle which would otherwise be deprived of blood and die (a myocardial infarct) when a major blood-vessel becomes occluded by a clot or by a fatty deposit in the wall of the artery. In other words, exercise is an insurance policy against a coronary thrombosis.

For a full discussion on the value of exercise, see Chapter 3. In the meanwhile, here are a few tips:

1 Avoid lifts and escalators whenever you can and walk up the stairs instead.

2 You should try to take sufficient exercise to get breathless sometime every day, and climbing stairs is a very good way.

3 Even if it is on an exercise bicycle while you are watching the television news, try and get a minimum of fifteen to twenty minutes exercise three times a week.

4 A brisk walk, perhaps to the shops and back, for a minimum of half an hour every day is also a very good exercise.

5 Whenever you can it is worth trying to make your housework routine into

exercises – stretching while doing the dusting; bending while doing the vacuum cleaning; pulling your abdominal muscles in ten times whenever you can remember.

There is a special regimen of exercises recommended by the Longevity Research Institute in California for people who suffer from heart disease. It involves a gradually increasing amount of exercise taken over a period of time – starting, say, with three short walks a day, becoming gradually longer until finally patients are able to go for a gentle jog. This routine has proved to be very successful in the rehabilitation of heart patients, and in helping those who are suffering from intermittent claudication (severe pain in the calves of the legs on walking due to an inadequate blood-supply to the muscles through narrowed arteries). Before undertaking such a regimen you should consult your doctor.

Smoking

The risk of heart disease among smokers is twice that among non-smokers. At the age of thirty-five it is four or five times higher. So if you have a tendency to develop heart disease, or if there are any members of your family who have developed heart disease, give up smoking if you possibly can. (For tips on how to control your smoking, see p. 77.)

One of the effects of nicotine is that it causes narrowing of the coronary vessels which supply the heart muscle with oxygen and nourishment. It follows that anyone who has a heart complaint of any kind such as high blood-pressure, or a condition affecting the blood-vessels such as narrowing of the arteries, is well advised not to smoke. It is mandatory that sufferers from angina should not smoke.

Stress

Stress is part and parcel of the 'businessman's disease' which, in the main, means heart disease. Heart disease is almost certainly linked with eating too much, drinking too much, smoking too much and not taking enough exercise. However, doctors are very familiar with the story that acute emotion of any kind, but particularly stress, may precipitate angina or a heart attack. And while we all must necessarily experience some stress in our lives, try to take steps to guard against being exposed to the worst of it and to learn to ameliorate the effects of it. It is worth trying to manage your life differently to avoid unnecessary or unproductive stress, and certainly to avoid exhaustion.

If you possibly can it is a very good idea to take up some method of relaxation – whatever suits you – be it yoga or transcendental meditation or simply teaching yourself to let each of the muscles in your body relax in turn by concentrating on the process of relaxation. It is important to get a good night's sleep and you will stand a better chance of getting it if you spend half an hour before going to bed trying to relax and wind down. Devise a going-to-bed-routine. Take a book to bed or watch television in bed if that is what you find soporific. At least once a week sleep late. Take turns with your husband or wife so that this lie-in is assured and you can catch up on lost rest. (See also **Insomnia**, pp. 177–8.)

We often feel more secure if we can assess a risk. You can estimate your chances of suffering heart disease by working out your score on the chart below, which was drawn up by the Michigan Heart Association. This chart puts together the various factors which are thought to affect one's predisposition to

Sex	**Systolic blood pressure** (Upper reading)	**Saturated fat in diet** (%)	**Exercise**
Female under 40 1	100 1	None 1	Intensive work and recreational exertion. 2
Female 40–50 2	120 2	10 2	Moderate work and recreational exertion. 2
Female 50+ 3	140 3	20 3	Sedentary work and intense recreational exertion. 3
Male 5	160 4	30 4	Sedentary work and moderate recreational exertion. 5
Stocky male 6	180 6	40 5	Sedentary work and light recreational exertion. 6
Bald stocky male 7	200 or over 8	50 7	Complete lack of exercise. 8

developing heart disease. Each of the factors is weighted and when these are added together they give a score which is the index of your risk. As you will see from the chart, it is better to be female than male (female hormones protect you from heart disease until after the menopause) and as you would expect, you are at less risk if you are underweight, if you don't smoke, if you take regular exercise and if your diet contains only a small amount of animal fat.

According to the Michigan Heart Association, the following scores indicate the risk of developing heart disease: 6–11: well below average; 12–17: below average; 18–24: average; 25–31: moderate; 32–40: dangerous; 41–63: imminent danger – see your doctor.

'After' Michigan Heart Association Chart

Tobacco smoking	**Weight**	**Heredity** (Family)	**Age**
Non-user. 0	More than 5 lb. below standard weight. 0	No known history of heart disease. 1	10–20 1
Cigar and or pipe (non-inhaling). 1	−5 lb. to +5 lb. standard weight. 1	One relative over sixty with cardiovascular disease. 2	21–30 2
Ten cigarettes or less a day. 2	0–20 lb. overweight. 2	Two relatives over sixty with cardiovascular disease. 4	31–40 3
Twenty cigarettes a day. 4	21–35 lb. overweight. 3	One relative under sixty with cardiovascular disease. 6	41–50 4
Thirty cigarettes a day. 6	36–50 lb. overweight. 5	Two relatives under sixty with cardiovascular disease. 6	51–60 5
Forty cigarettes a day or more. 10	51–65 lb. overweight. 7	Three relatives under sixty with cardiovascular disease. 7	61–70 8

5 Having a Healthy Chest

Having a healthy chest is not entirely in your hands. While your mother is carrying you in pregnancy her habits can affect the health of your lungs. If your mother smokes, for instance, she is increasing the risk of you being born with respiratory disease of the newborn. This condition is not completely understood, but a newborn baby suffering from it breathes inefficiently and erratically. More seriously, the immature lungs perform the job of gaseous exchange imperfectly, so that in the early days of life such a baby may suffer from a relative lack of oxygen. Babies of mothers who smoke in pregnancy are also predisposed to chest infections and to sudden cot death. If you are a woman and become pregnant, the least you can do for your baby is to give up smoking, and by doing so bequeath to your child a healthy pair of lungs with which to start its life.

How childhood ailments affect the chest in later life

Reaching adulthood with undamaged lungs is like picking your way through a minefield because several diseases of childhood can leave their mark on the lungs into later life. The two most serious infectious childhood diseases from the point of view of permanent damage to the lungs are whooping cough and measles.

Whooping cough inflicts most damage on the lungs during the first year of life. Breast-fed babies, however, are protected while being breast-fed because they take in antibodies to whooping cough with their mother's milk. This is not so with bottle-fed babies. Therefore it is particularly important to protect these babies from whooping cough by having them immunized. (For discussion on whooping cough immunization see pp. 78–9.)

The whooping cough germ viciously attacks the lung which becomes inflamed and produces large quantities of mucus to protect itself. When the inflammation heals it may leave scars which distort the tiny, fragile air sacs, and some of the natural elasticity of the lung is destroyed. One of the narrow air passages may become completely blocked so that the lung behind the blockage collapses. Thereafter there is always the danger of infection occurring in the collapsed lung, and, should this occur, your child may be left with bronchiectasis – a chronic infection of the lung which can follow on from the destruction of lung tissues such as occurs in whooping cough. Antibiotics are frequently ineffective because they cannot penetrate to the infection. The condition obviously lowers the efficiency of the lungs and sufferers may get short of breath on exercise. They may appear a little blue around the mouth because the blood cannot be fully oxygenated in the infected lungs (see p. 20). Due to modern treatment this is now a rare complication of whooping cough, fortunately so because it is a constant drain on the child's well-being, requiring rigorous medical attention and regular physiotherapy. These changes may leave the lungs permanently weakened with predisposition to infection.

Measles is a very virulent virus which can affect the ear and the brain (producing meningitis), the eye and the chest. The virus itself is responsible for a primary illness which can involve the chest in the same way as whooping cough. Additionally, it can weaken the lungs and the body's resistance to such an extent that the lungs become infected with secondary invaders – bacteria. This can lead to the development of pneumonia and serious respiratory distress which, in a small child, may require hospitalization. A severe attack of pneumonia may leave a young child with a permanently damaged lung. The immunization regimen can protect babies from measles as well so the importance of adhering to it cannot be over-emphasized.

In small children the respiratory passages are small and therefore easily blocked by secretions. This means that if an infection settles in one part, it can quickly travel to another. In a young child, therefore, sinusitis may develop very rapidly into bronchitis and a cold may spread to become an infected middle ear. Consequently doctors are used to considering the sinuses, the nose, the ears, the throat, the bronchial tubes and the chest as one system in children. For this reason they tend to treat an infection in one part of the respiratory passages very strenuously to prevent it involving another. This is particularly true if the child has a recurrent condition. Recurrent sinusitis can quickly become chronic bronchitis, as can recurrent middle-ear infections. In young children it is important to treat sinusitis, middle-ear infections and tonsillitis promptly to prevent the development of chronic bronchitis which may stay with the child into later life.

Good and bad breathing

The lungs are a pair of beautifully designed, very efficient bellows with the approximate surface area of a tennis court (see pp. 18–20). The mechanical function of the lungs is to get air in and out, but as most of us are lazy, air probably comes in contact with no more than two-thirds of the surface area of the lungs. Most of us take shallow breaths most of the time and never aerate the lower parts of the lung, which are well down at waist level, other than on those rare occasions when we fling open the window and gulp half a dozen deep breaths. So most of the time our lungs are being used well below their capacity. This is due to a variety of factors, including bad posture which tends to confine the lungs, sedentary jobs, which do not involve physical activity or allow full expansion of the chest; and tight clothes, which can limit the respiratory excursion of the chest wall.

The act of taking a breath in has two components. The first is due to the expansion of the chest wall upwards and outwards by the muscles between the ribs, and the second is due to the compression of the abdomen downwards and outwards by the relaxation of the diaphragm. The reverse happens when a breath is exhaled. In Victorian times when tight corsets were the fashion, the constriction of the whalebone prevented the abdominal element of inspiration and women relied entirely on the chest component. Many of them were probably living in a permanent state of partial oxygen starvation, which may account for their frequent attacks of the vapours.

Breathing exercises are rarely necessary if one is performing any type of regular exercise. The sort of exercises you should be doing to keep fit (see pp. 59–64) involve going on until you are short of breath; this in itself is sufficient to expand the lungs to their full capacity.

Coughs and colds

The cough reflex is essential to the maintenance of a healthy chest. Coughing is a very efficient way of getting rid of mucus which has been cleared from the lungs to the back of the throat. There it produces an irritation which results in an explosive exhalation of air during which the air may travel at more than one hundred miles an hour.

A productive cough, that is one which is producing sputum, is performing such a useful function that it should never be suppressed. Despite the discomfort and the possibility of restless nights, it is better to 'cough up the phlegm' than to leave it in the lungs and have a full night's sleep. You can help to ease a night cough by using three or four pillows and by sleeping on your side. Only a dry cough which is not producing sputum should be suppressed.

When I was a little girl there was a saying in our part of the world that when the mucus from a cold or cough turned yellow then it was getting better. In one way this is true. Yellow mucus from the sinuses, nose or chest is pus, and it means that an infection is present. Although the cold is worse the time to recovery is shorter in the purulent stage than in the catarrhal stage. Mucus from a virus infection is nearly always thin, colourless and watery, but it becomes thick and yellowy green when bacterial infection is superimposed. Yellow mucus and sputum must always have medical treatment, usually in the form of antibiotics. As soon as you notice the colour change in mucus from the nose or chest, consult your doctor. Because of their relationship to chronic bronchitis, sinus infections and bronchitis should always be taken seriously.

Smoking and chronic bronchitis

The association between smoking and the development of lung cancer and heart disease are discussed elsewhere (see pp. 94–5 and p. 69), but just as important is the connection between smoking and the development of chronic bronchitis. Chronic bronchitis is a common but serious disease. In 1975 it claimed nearly thirty thousand lives and was responsible for the loss of almost ten million working days in the United Kingdom. Working in dusty environments is a causative factor in a small proportion of cases, but far and away the most important cause is cigarette smoking.

Cigarette smoking is irritating. Some smokers and all non-smokers have experienced a stinging in the eyes when they are sitting in a room full of cigarette smoke. The stinging is caused by the noxious chemicals in cigarette smoke. When we inhale cigarette smoke into our lungs all the bronchial passages are irritated in the same way as our eyes. Our eyes respond by watering and become red. Our lungs respond by producing excessive quantities of mucus in an attempt to bathe the inflamed membranes with a soothing balm. But as we shall see, this turns out to be a hindrance not a help.

An additional effect of the chemicals in cigarette smoke is to damage the cilia which line the bronchial passages. Cilia are tiny hairs which cover the membranes inside the bronchial tubes in their millions. They are in constant movement. They waft upwards and their job is to carry foreign particles and mucus up to the back of the throat. When sufficient mucus collects there you are stimulated to cough and expel the debris to the outside. The effect of cigarette smoke is to diminish the mobility of the cilia. Consequently mucus and debris from the inside of the lungs is not removed efficiently and may stagnate, becoming ripe for infection should it strike, as it does every winter in the form of influenza. Mentholated cigarettes, contrary to the medicinal and health-giving aura they have attracted, damage the cilia even more. Menthol may paralyse them altogether.

So far we have three deleterious effects of cigarette smoking: it produces an irritation to the lining of the lungs which leads to the production of excess quantities of mucus; this excess mucus may pool and become the medium in which viruses or bacteria grow; the clearing action of the cilia in the lungs is interfered with. Symptoms which go hand in hand with these effects are: a chronic cough (due to excess mucus), particularly first thing in the morning when the overnight mucus has pooled in the bronchial tubes; head colds always seem to go to the chest; and a tendency to develop bronchitic conditions. These symptoms herald the onset of chronic bronchitis.

Chronic bronchitis traditionally goes through the following steps:

1 Intermittent cough which never clears completely.

2 Cough throughout most of the winter.

3 Winter cold or flu that develops into bronchitis.

4 Three or four attacks of cold, sinusitis or flu in a year which all develop into chronic bronchitis.

5 Diminishing periods of freedom between attacks of bronchitis in the winter.

6 Bronchitis all the way through the winter.

7 Attacks of bronchitis during the summer too.

By the time this happens your breathing will have been seriously impaired. You will get short of breath when you run for a bus or when you try to climb a flight of stairs at speed or when you carry bags any distance. Your sputum, which was once whitish or greyish, will now be almost permanently yellowish or greenish. This means that it is infected. It means that the inside of your lungs is never free of grumbling suppuration. This is not only bad for your breathing, it is also a drain on your general good health and it weakens your defences in resisting other diseases.

The intermittent attacks of chronic inflammation in your lung heal with scarring and this distorts the natural architecture of the lung. Gradually the air spaces are broken down and the lung loses its elasticity and the ability to recoil. The first thing that you will notice is difficulty in breathing out: you can breathe in but it requires a lot of effort to breathe out. With each intake of breath the lungs become slightly more expanded but they cannot be emptied and eventually your lungs will be in a state of permanent semi-expansion. Of course, this is very detrimental to gaseous exchange which is the chemical function of the lungs. The lungs can no longer provide oxygen to the rest of the body and the means by which the body can get rid of carbon dioxide. Because the level of oxygen in your blood remains low the blood is not fully oxygenated and your skin takes on a bluish tinge.

By this time the chronic bronchitis has progressed to a condition called emphysema which, at its worst, is a crippling disease. Shortness of breath restricts almost all physical movement to a degree which may necessitate confinement to a chair or bed. Every breath becomes a physical struggle.

Asthma may become superimposed on chronic bronchitis or emphysema at any time and this greatly worsens the outlook. For besides having to deal with chronically inflamed, infected and damaged lungs, asthma gives the patient the added burden of having to breathe through constricted bronchial tubes.

It seems hard to imagine that all this can start with a furtive cigarette behind the school bicycle shed. Good advice would be to eschew smoking at any cost and, if you do smoke, do your utmost to give it up by whatever means you can. In a recent newspaper article, six people described their experiences in trying to give up smoking; only two succeeded. One of those who failed said that he would have had a better chance of success if he had had a dramatic health reason for giving up smoking.

If you must smoke try to follow these guidelines:

1 Always smoke cigarettes with a filter.

2 Always smoke low-tar cigarettes.

3 Smoke less than five cigarettes a day if you possibly can.

4 Do not inhale.

5 Throw away a long stub.

6 Do not offer cigarettes to your friends.

7 Do not smoke in front of children.

8 Try switching to cigars or a pipe but do not inhale those either.

9 Keep cigarettes as far away from you as possible so that getting one involves the maximum effort.

6 Preventive Medicine

Infectious diseases

You may have been the beneficiary of preventive medicine earlier in your life than you think. If your mother opted to breast feed you, you had a flying start from day one because she was practising her own special brand of preventive medicine on your behalf. Colostrum and breast milk contain the antibodies to all the infections that your mother had ever contracted. She passed these on to you when she breast fed you. What is more, you were protected against all the diseases to which she had developed antibodies for as long as she breast fed you.

Breast feeding confers *passive* immunity on the baby, and while it serves the baby very well in the first few months of life, the best preventive medicine confers *active* immunity to infections. In passive immunity, antibodies are absorbed into the body. Active immunity involves the production of antibodies by the body's own defence mechanisms. The body can be stimulated to produce antibodies by injecting small quantities of dead or weakened germs which the body can recognize as foreign. The response is to produce antibodies to kill them. This exposure to foreign germs 'primes' our defence mechanisms so that the body is always in a state of preparedness should it meet that germ again. Passive immunity lasts a matter of days or weeks. Active immunity lasts for years. Nonetheless it usually needs boosting and, as with tetanus, you should be reimmunized every three years or so.

Active immunity is conferred by immunization. It is possible to be actively immunized against quite a number of diseases including diphtheria, whooping cough, tetanus, polio (infantile paralysis), measles, German measles, smallpox, tuberculosis, typhoid, cholera and yellow fever. By assiduously following immunization regimens against these infections, most of them can be prevented.

Immunization should start early in life but not too early. Babies usually begin their immunization scheme at the age of three months. Injections and polio drops are given according to the schedule described below:

1 Triple injections at three, four and six months (diphtheria, whooping cough, tetanus) and diphtheria and tetanus pre-school.

2 Poliomyelitis drops at three, four and six months and pre-school.

3 Measles during second year (single injection).

4 BCG (anti-tuberculosis) offered between the ages of ten and thirteen if testing shows they have no immunity.

5 Smallpox.

6 German measles (rubella) at about twelve, to girls.

Smallpox and tetanus need a booster every three years. Typhoid, types A and B, the so-called TAB injection, needs revaccination after a similar time.

Whether or not to give a baby whooping cough vaccine still remains, at the time of writing, a controversy. Results of surveys of infants vaccinated against whooping cough, previously unreported, do record a few cases of brain damage after the vaccination. On the credit side, significantly fewer of the children vaccinated suffered severe whooping cough. You must weigh against the statistics on brain damage from vaccination the fact that a few children who contract whooping cough also get brain damage. Furthermore, we know that if the proportion of vaccinated children falls below a certain level there can be epidemics of whooping cough. Vaccination, therefore, protects the community as well as your baby. In general, most doctors would be in favour of vaccination but all parents should be told of signs to look out for after the first of the three injections. Their appearance contraindicates subsequent injections. Report any of these to your doctor immediately: a very high temperature within forty-eight hours, large swelling at the site of the injection, vomiting, or a convulsion.

The protection from both cholera and yellow fever injections is fairly short-lived, probably only six to nine months. You should therefore probably have a booster injection whenever you are travelling to countries where these diseases are endemic (enquire of the appropriate embassy in London if in doubt), especially if it is six months since you had a vaccination. Always check with your doctor if you are unsure.

Medicine has not found a way to confer active immunity against malaria. However it is possible to practise preventive medicine against it. Whenever you are travelling to a malarious area you should ask your doctor for a supply of anti-malarial drugs to take prophylactically to protect you against malarial infection. Whenever you are in a malarious area you should take your malaria prophylaxis religiously.

Teeth

Fashions in dentistry have changed markedly over the last few decades. At one time it was thought fashionable, to some it was even a status symbol, to have all the teeth removed and false teeth fitted. This was particularly prevalent in the north of England and Scotland. The lower social groups in particular opted for the fashion, and men more than women. Even today, nine million teeth are extracted every year and another thirty-six million are filled. Dental decay is the commonest disease affecting us today, with over thirty-five per cent of people over sixteen having none of their teeth left at all. Dental statistics are staggering: seven out of ten children entering school have tooth decay; four out of every five eight-year-olds need treatment; only five per cent of teenagers in school are free of dental decay. The tide of fashion however has turned. The motto now is '*Preserve teeth at all costs*', which means '*Prevent dental decay at all costs*'.

Inherited weaknesses of the teeth aside, we know that the major causes of caries are the cumulative effects of a sweet starchy diet and poor personal dental care. Any sweet food, including sweet drinks, encourages dental decay. Comforters containing sweet drinks should be avoided. Dentists recognize the total destruction of teeth that this causes as 'bottle mouth'. Even some drinks which mothers give in their children's best interest are bad for their teeth – for instance, fruit juices, particularly blackcurrant juice. Other sweet things which inflict damage are mint sweets and cola drinks. A mother has two options to combat the effect of sweet food on her children's teeth: she can either ban them or she can take precautions to prevent the harm that they cause. One of the ways of doing the latter is to make sure that your children always brush their teeth immediately after taking a sweet drink, or sucking a sweet, or eating sweet foods and always, always before they go to bed at night.

Professional dental care should always start from an early age. All of my children, invariably accompanied by their elder siblings, have visited the dentist quite painlessly [*sic!*] from the age of two and a half. Checks should be at least every six months. So that your children will remember visits to the dentist with pleasure try to find a dentist in your area who specializes in the dental care of children.

Despite controversy, a report from the Royal College of Physicians came out in favour of fluoride supplements to prevent tooth decay in children. If you live in an area where the fluoridation of water supplies has not taken place, you can give fluoride tablets to your children as an alternative. Fluoride tablets, which are available from most chemist shops, should be given as soon as a child is capable of swallowing them up to the age of eleven when the second teeth are normally fully formed. This alone would cut the incidence of dental decay by as much as half.

Many a dentist, on looking into a mouth, feels like saying: 'Well, your teeth are all right but your gums will have to come out.' Without healthy gums your teeth are in danger, no matter how healthy they are. The health of your gums is endangered mainly by the formation of plaque. Plaque forms as a deposit from saliva plus sugars and proteins from the bacteria themselves. If plaque is not removed it collects in the crevices between the teeth and is converted to a hard chalky substance which extends down into the spaces between the teeth and the gums. It causes inflammation of the gum margins and pockets form in the gums around the teeth. In these pockets bacteria collect and multiply and a chronic grumbling infection is set up. Teeth become loose in the mouth as the gum recedes. The final stage is pyorrhoea. Severe pyorrhoea is almost impossible to eradicate and very often the only cure is removal of all the teeth.

The formation of plaque is diminished by eating a correct diet. It is prevented from collecting by brushing properly and by the use of dental floss. You cannot brush your teeth effectively unless you have a good toothbrush, so here are some of the criteria to remember when you are choosing a new one:

1 All the bristles should be the same length – leave serrated toothbrushes on the chemist's shelf.

2 Nylon bristles are better than pure bristles which tend to split.

3 The toothbrush should be medium soft.

4 You should replace your toothbrush every month at least.

5 Always brush your teeth with a vertical movement, down for upper teeth and up for lower teeth.

If your children are taking fluoride tablets, make sure they chew them up because fluoride has a local protective effect as well as an inner one. Toothpastes which do not contain fluoride are purely cosmetic, the only advantage they have is that they make the operation of brushing your teeth more pleasant. You should avoid especially formulated children's toothpastes with flavours; these are really a contradiction in terms because they sometimes contain sugar. Check the ingredients before buying, and, if they are not stated, do not buy. Adults, too, benefit from using fluoride toothpastes.

Feet

The feet deserve special mention. Being the furthest distance away from the heart, they are the least well nourished part of the body. Being dependent, waste materials and water tend to pool there, especially as we age; the blood takes longer to reach the feet and impurities have to fight their way against the force of gravity to be removed. That is why any small infection or injury to the feet takes longer to heal than anywhere else in the body. If you have an injury to the foot you can speed up recovery by raising the feet whenever you sit or lie down, thereby promoting drainage of the blood from your feet. Elastic stockings can also act as a support and an artificial pump to keep the blood circulating efficiently.

All our weight is supported by our feet and so, despite their fairly small size and comparatively delicate structure, they are under great strain. It follows that

Contraceptive	Mechanism of action	Effectiveness (pregnancies per 100 women years)
IUD	Any foreign body in the womb will prevent conception.	3
DIAPHRAGM	Prevents sperm reaching the womb.	2–3
SHEATH	Prevents sperm being deposited in the vagina.	4
VASECTOMY	Sperm cannot reach the penis because tubes carrying them are cut.	0
STERILIZATION	Fallopian tubes cut so egg cannot reach womb.	0
COMBINED PILL	Prevents ovulation.	Less than 1

Contraception table

we should not abuse them with ill-fitting shoes, with hazardous shoe design (for example, platform-soled shoes which can strain the feet sufficiently to cause fracture of the bones), and we should pay special care and attention to calluses, corns, ingrowing toenails, bunions and the like. Perhaps only toothache is worse than sore feet, so it is worth taking care of yours from early in life. (See also **Feet complaints**, p. 167.)

Family planning

Family planning means spacing your children, limiting the number of children you have or deciding not to have any at all. With the advent of family planning clinics, advice on contraception is available which enables you to space your family as you wish. The factors which affect your decision will naturally include socio-economic ones, but important new research should make us consider longer gaps between our children. It has shown that the longer the time a child spends as 'the baby' of the family, the better he or she will thrive, physically, emotionally and intellectually.

Most family planning clinics and family planning doctors can provide you with a wide range of contraceptive methods on which they will give advice so that you are able to take advantage of the one which best suits you and your spouse. The efficacy of any method of contraception depends very much on the

Pros	Cons	Comments
Can be left for two years.	May be painful and periods can be heavy.	Have it fitted at a family planning clinic if possible.
No physical side effects.	Unaesthetic.	Use with spermicidal cream or foam.
No physical side effects.	Unaesthetic.	Use with spermicidal cream or foam.
Does not affect male libido.	Irreversible.	It takes three to four months for sperm to disappear so take extra precautions for this time.
Pregnancy is impossible.	Irreversible.	Menstruation may be irregular after operation.
Easy to take. Aesthetic.	Reported side effects.	Regular medical supervision needed.

diligence of the person using it. The pill used carelessly can have a higher failure rate than the diaphragm used meticulously.

The decision to take an oral contraceptive involves special preventive medicine measures. Oral contraceptives containing female hormones should always be considered as *medicines* and should never be taken without your doctor's supervision and without regular medical check-ups. When you go on the pill you will probably be asked to attend a medical check at six weeks and then at three months, then possibly at six months and again at a year. After that, annual check-ups are probably sufficient but your doctor will advise you how often you should have them.

At each visit the following checks will probably be done: weight gain; urine testing; blood-pressure reading; smear testing (usually annually); examination of legs for varicose veins; and examination of the breasts.

While you are on an oral contraceptive any pains in the chest or a sudden attack of breathlessness should prompt you to seek medical advice. If you have had a thrombosis in the past you are not a suitable person to take the pill.

Here are some of the more important things that you should know before you start taking the pill. This list is not supposed to be exhaustive. Full information can be obtained from your doctor (and make sure you have all your questions answered) or from the manufacturer's literature.

1 You should take the pill only if your physician definitely says that you *can*. You should not take it in these conditions:

(a) If you have a history of high blood-pressure, a stroke, a clot on the lung, or infection or clotting of varicose veins.
(b) If you have liver disease, or jaundice, or severe itching during pregnancy.
(c) If you have had any abnormal bleeding of which the cause was not found.
(d) If you suspect you are pregnant.
(e) If you are breast feeding; small amounts of contraceptives have been found in mothers' milk, but the effect on infants is not known. You may experience reduction of your milk supply.

2 Before you go on to the pill make sure you tell your doctor if you are taking any medicines regularly such as sleeping tablets or antibiotics or medicines used in the treatment of epilepsy or tuberculosis.

3 Menstruation should be fully established before taking the pill.

4 Bleeding: slight spotting between periods while on the pill is normally not something to worry about. If bleeding persists medical advice should be sought.

5 Vaginal irritation or discharge: you should go and see your doctor if any vaginal irritation or discharge occurs because this may be due to an overgrowth of a yeast-type germ which can be readily treated.

6 Surgery: if you need an operation or have to go into hospital as an emergency, inform your hospital doctor that you are taking a contraceptive.

Pregnancy

Nowadays preventive medicine in the form of early and regular ante-natal care is widely practised in pregnancy. For instance, all pregnant women routinely receive iron supplements and one of the B vitamins – folic acid – as soon as pregnancy is diagnosed, because there is a natural tendency in pregnancy to become anaemic due to iron deficiency and folic acid deficiency. To feed the growing baby, extra amounts of vitamins and minerals are needed and milk is one of the best sources of these foods. So pregnant mothers are encouraged to drink a pint of milk a day. If you hate milk your baby will not suffer as long as you take some dairy products each day.

By giving up smoking you can decrease the chance of your child having difficulty with breathing when it is born and the possibility of it being stillborn.

During the first three months of pregnancy you should take no drugs whatsoever, except under medical supervision. While most drugs are intensively tested for their potential to affect an early developing foetus, it is good medical practice to avoid drugs in the early stages of pregnancy.

With the advent of amniocentesis doctors can learn things about the unborn baby that makes possible a new kind of preventive medicine. Amniocentesis is a simple surgical manoeuvre whereby a specimen of the fluid surrounding the developing baby can be drawn off and examined in a laboratory. It is a minor procedure but it has its hazards, for example, infection, and so it should not be considered lightly. There are certain circumstances where it can be very helpful to doctors. Amniocentesis may be used to help in the diagnosis of rare neonatal disorders, but there are two fairly common disorders in which it can be illuminating. These are mongolism and spinabifida.

Mongolism is most common when either, or both, of the parents are old. In such a situation a specimen of the amniotic fluid may be removed and by very careful examination under a microscope the chromosomes in the cells of the baby can be examined. Mongolism, an abnormality of the chromosomes, can then be picked up.

Spina bifida runs in families and there are grounds for performing amniocentesis in any mother who has previously given birth to a child suffering from spina bifida or if any of her relatives have suffered from the disease. The diagnosis is made by the finding of an abnormal protein in the amniotic fluid. If mongolism and spina bifida are confirmed, both parents are usually told and are given the option to make a decision for the mother to have an early abortion.

Any pregnant woman should watch out for the following signs and draw her doctor's attention to them immediately should they appear:

1 Swelling of the ankles.
2 Rings that become tight on the fingers.
3 'Show' of blood from the vagina.
4 The appearance of varicose veins.
5 The appearance of piles.
6 Frequent severe headaches.
7 Loss of consciousness or fainting.
8 Shortness of breath.
9 Palpitations.
10 Itching of the genital organs.
11 Burning sensation when passing urine.
12 Any rash.

Pre-menstrual tension

Very few women are entirely free of symptoms during the week prior to menstruation, and possibly during the first few days of menstruation. Symptoms can vary from headaches, backache, joint pains, irritability, tearfulness, insomnia to much more serious illnesses like worsening of asthma, migraine, epilepsy, and to psychological disturbances which can injure the health and happiness of the family and marriage.

Dr Katharina Dalton has done a great deal of research which clarifies our thinking and our understanding of this very real and occasionally serious event which punctuates a woman's life at monthly intervals. Not only has she found that women who suffer from pre-menstrual tension are more likely to commit crimes at this time, are more likely to have accidents, are more susceptible to the effects of alcohol, and will drink more alcohol, but that they are more inclined to batter their children. In many instances, perfectly normal happy women, with a usual sunny disposition, can change their personalities so that they become almost unrecognizable to their own families.

Dr Dalton advocates, and has indeed found, that treatment with progesterone can well nigh eradicate the symptoms of pre-menstrual tension and in many cases bring relief from the monthly exacerbations of illness like asthma. She has found the most successful way of giving the progesterone is in the form of an implant. Under local anaesthetic a small incision is made in the skin and a pellet is inserted under the skin. The pellet slowly releases its progesterone over a period of time.

The retention of water is thought to contribute to pre-menstrual tension and some women have recorded huge increases in weight, as much as 14 lb., but increases of between 5–7 lb. are fairly common – all of which is lost in a few days after menstruation begins. If this applies to you then your symptoms might be helped by the use of diuretics. These drugs, which eliminate water from the body, are only available on prescriptions, and would only be given to you if your doctor felt that they would be useful. (See also **Pre-menstrual tension**, pp. 190–1.)

The menopause

While treatments have been on trial over the years for the treatment of menopausal symptoms, including sedatives, tranquillizers, sleeping pills, vitamin courses, iron therapy, and many forms of psychotherapy, it has been found that some menopausal symptoms, such as hot flushes, depression and loss of sex drive, can be alleviated by the cyclical administration of hormone preparations containing oestrogen and progestogen. Recent medical research has concluded that it is necessary to give progestogen, along with oestrogen, for at least thirteen days each month as this helps to guard against the excessive build-up of the lining of the womb by producing a regular monthly bleed.

Professor Christopher Nordin from Leeds has shown unequivocally that the administration of female hormones to menopausal women can prevent osteoporosis, or softening of the bone, and can arrest it if it has already begun. His research has also shown that over the age of sixty-five it is not hormones which protect the bones but vitamin D. He therefore recommends that vitamin D supplements and calcium are given to all women over the age of sixty-five. (See also **Menopause**, pp. 181–2.)

Venereal disease

Not only is the incidence of venereal disease increasing but, more seriously, the bacteria which cause venereal disease are becoming resistant to traditional forms of antibiotic therapy. It is therefore essential that venereal disease is contained and prevented. This can mainly be done by counselling and publicity and most importantly, by a responsible attitude to teenage sex in parents and teachers. Early in their lives children should be told, most appropriately at school, that disease can be transmitted during sexual intercourse. The signs and symptoms of these diseases should be fully explained so that youngsters will be alert to their appearance. The immediate and long-term dangers of venereal disease should be explained in full. Most teenage girls who learn that sterility or infertility is a common consequence of venereal disease should find that fact alone a sufficient deterrent to promiscuity. Teenagers should be told where and how they can seek confidential help and a responsible attitude to pre-marital sex and venereal disease should be encouraged so that if a disease is detected or suspected, it is not knowingly spread. (See also **Venereal diseases**, pp. 201.)

Routine medical checks

As a general rule routine medical checks are not advocated as their disadvantages frequently outweigh their advantages. Many otherwise unworried people may be unnecessarily frightened by a finding which to a doctor is of little significance. Obsessiveness with health can also lead to hypochondria. A general rule for medical checks is that you should not opt to have one until you feel you have the need for one, *and then always consult your doctor first.*

However, there are certain medical checks which probably should be performed at regular intervals throughout your life to pick up preventable conditions or to prevent minor defects from becoming serious problems. Such checks would include:

1 Mammography of the breast for the early detection of a breast tumour.

2 Cervical smear test for the early detection of changes in the cells of the cervix.

3 Mass miniature radiography (MMR) for the detection of pulmonary tuberculosis and lung tumours.

4 Routine eye tests of children before they go to school.

5 Routine eye tests of adults over the age of fifty for the detection of glaucoma which is responsible for one in ten cases of blindness in adults.

6 General practitioners to examine, where possible, all adults for the detection of high blood-pressure.

7 Detailed 'business men and women's checks' which can be performed at special clinics. They should include a full haematological and biochemical examination, full medical and laboratory checks on cardiac, liver and kidney function. These checks are available either through your own doctor or through insurance companies, but they should not be undertaken without consulting your own doctor first.

7 Cancer

The following chapter is written in the belief that the more we know, the more we can help ourselves. No alarmism is intended; the approach is straightforward and honest.

As often as not it is we who allow cancer to kill us. Nearly all cancers treated early enough are curable. The sad fact is that most patients with cancer only seek treatment at a late stage in the development of the tumour when the possibility of a cure is greatly diminished.

There are several reasons for this. Firstly, most people are not aware of symptoms which are suggestive of the presence of early cancer and therefore do not heed warning signs which should take them to their doctor. Secondly, many are fearful of cancer and fearful of having their worst suspicions confirmed by their doctor. So they procrastinate and by the time they consult their doctor the chance of a cure is slight.

The popular concept of cancer is a mysterious dreadful disease which is almost always fatal. This idea has caused an almost superstitious fear. Unfortunately the general public know very little about the large number of patients who have been successfully treated and who are living out their normal lifespan with no trouble and no sign of recurrence. Almost all of these patients sought treatment at an early stage of their disease and it is therefore important to correct the phobia that surrounds cancer. People must understand that there are real chances of curing cancers. This will help to eradicate the irrational fear which causes delay in seeking medical advice and consequent delay in diagnosis. It is important for the medical profession to undertake education campaigns which will lead to a better understanding and to freedom from inaccurate and traditional beliefs. Dr Maurice Sutton of the Tenovus Cancer Information Centre in Wales has made concerted efforts to disseminate accurate details about cancer. A particularly good review is a booklet entitled *Cancer Explained* by Dr Sutton (Evans Bros., London).

What is cancer?

Despite the fact that we still have not discovered the cause of cancer, much is known about other aspects of the disease and we have accumulated a great deal of experience in the vigorous and successful treatment of it. First of all, what is cancer? Cancer in simple terms is an abnormal growth of cells. It usually starts with the abnormal growth of a single cell. This abnormally growing cell can reproduce itself and form two abnormally growing cells. This pair can reproduce themselves to give four, thence eight, sixteen, thirty-two, sixty-four, until there are a large number of cancerous cells growing in one spot. Eventually the cells give rise to a lump or tumour. Under normal circumstances cell growth is controlled so that cells reproduce themselves only at a rate fast enough to replace cells which are dying. In cancer, cell growth is no longer under normal control. Cells grow at a haphazard rate and at the expense of the parent organ.

We witness every day examples of the normal control of cell growth. For instance, if we cut ourselves the cut in the skin is healed by the formation of a scar and the scar tissue does not extend beyond the edges of the cut. Repair (cell growth) is controlled. If we break a bone, the bone ends heal through the production of new bone, but the new bone cells do not spread beyond the boundaries of the break. There appears to be some police force which keeps the cell population in order. This police force has been called the 'organizer'. It is fairly obvious that in cancer, organizers can no longer control the rate of cell growth, or they no longer exist, or they are neutralized by another force. Any cell in the body can become independent of its organizer. It follows that a cancer can grow in any sort of tissue. If a breast cell is affected, then breast cancer develops; if a skin cell is affected, skin cancer results; if a lung cell is affected, bronchial cancer will form.

Cancer cells have several characteristics which distinguish them immediately from normal slow-growing cells. If they are examined under the microscope they appear to be 'busy'. They are rather irregular in shape and disorganized in arrangement. The central nucleus which controls most of the cell's activity is larger and darker than usual. Cancer cells also have the ability to spread. They invade surrounding tissues. They can break off and float via the blood-stream to other parts of the body and produce 'metastases'. Cancer of the stomach will produce mestastases in the liver, cancer of the breast will metastasize to the brain. The consistency of cancer cells is usually different from normal tissue and if a breast cancer is cut through, the tumour is of a harder, grittier consistency than normal breast tissue.

So it can be seen that cancer is a disturbance of normal cell growth. Most tumours consisting of abnormally growing cells are not cancer. The majority of them are benign and cause no harmful effect to the patient, nor do they spread to other parts of the body. So a benign tumour of the skin produces a lump only in the skin, while a malignant tumour of the skin will produce a lump in the skin but its cells may spread to other distant parts of the body. Benign tumours are much more common than cancerous tumours though sometimes it is difficult for doctors to distinguish between them simply by feeling them. They can however be easily separated by examining them under a microscope. Benign tumours are so common that it is very rare to see someone who has none and they are, in the main, of very little importance.

Quite often a cancerous tumour is growing so fast that it outgrows the supply of nourishment brought to it via the blood and the centre of it may die and form an ulcer. Remember that an ulcer to a doctor is merely a description of what he can see, i.e. a broken surface with an infected or dead central area; it is not a specific diagnosis. So just as there are benign and malignant tumours there are also benign and malignant ulcers.

Factors associated with the development of cancer

While the precise cause of cancer is not known, a great deal of research is being done to try to discover it and intensive detective work continues in research centres throughout the world. So far we know that there are four very important factors which are involved with the development of cancer. They are viruses, chemicals, atomic radiation and geographical or environmental factors.

Viruses are so small that they cannot be seen under an ordinary microscope and scientists are divided as to whether they are living or non-living. They reproduce themselves, which is a property possessed only by living things, but they are capable of very little else. What is more, they can only reproduce themselves inside living cells. Scientists feel that if viruses are the cause of cancer then it should be possible to infect an animal with cancer by injecting it with extracts from malignant tumours from another animal. Research done on rabbits has shown that this is possible and the virus is similar to the one that causes myxomatosis. There is also one transmissible cancer which is induced by a virus and affects fowl, but as far as we know, human cancer is not infectious. It was only at the beginning of this century that scientists first realized that tumours could be associated with chemicals. This was noticed when workers in the dye industry developed tumours of the bladder. The offending chemical was later found to be a substance called beta-methylamine. If you are exposed to this chemical the chances of developing bladder cancer are sixty times greater than if you are not.

In the nineteenth century it was noticed that men working on cotton-spinning machines developed cancer of the scrotum. Much later the cancer-producing substance was found in the mineral oil which was used to lubricate the machines and which splashed on to the workers' clothes and tended to collect around the scrotal area.

Then in 1916 two Japanese scientists started some experiments in which they regularly painted the skin of rabbits with tar over a period of several months. Cancer developed at the site where the tar had been applied. In 1933 the chemical in tar which had induced the cancer was identified as 3.4-benzpyrene. That 3.4-benzpyrene is found in cigarette smoke, provides one of the strongest arguments in support of cigarette smoking being associated with lung cancer. The statistics on this association have been and will be long argued but the association itself seems to be incontrovertible. There is no doubt that people who stop smoking have a lower risk of developing lung cancer than those who do not.

Ever since the early workers with X-rays developed cancer of the hands, atomic radiation has been known to be carcinogenic (induces cancer) and much evidence in favour of this theory has accumulated. In the early 1920s girls working in a New Jersey luminous paint factory developed bone cancer. It was discovered that they were licking their paint brushes to bring them to a fine point and in doing this they swallowed paint which contained radioactive radium. This radioactive chemical concentrated in bone, thereby delivering a high dose of radiation and this eventually led to the development of bone cancer.

Since the sixteenth century it has been known that certain ore miners suffer from a chest disease which only later was found to be cancer of the lung. The particular mines contained many radioactive ores and the air in the mines was full of radon, a radioactive dust. It is probable that the lung cancer was caused by continuously breathing the radioactive gases which contaminated the air inside the mines.

Scientists have noted that the incidence of different cancers is different in different parts of the world and in different races. Thus liver cancer is very rare in Western Europe but is the commonest form of cancer in Africa. Breast cancer is almost unheard of in Japan but very common in the United Kingdom and the U.S.A. Cancer of the nose is one of the most common to be found in China but is very rare in the western world. There are many theories explaining this, some have a firmer basis than others. Skin cancer, for instance, is common in Australia and this is probably due to the number of hours of ultraviolet radiation (sunlight) to which Australians are exposed. It is possible that liver cancer in Africans is connected with their poor diet which is almost bereft of the vitamins necessary for the health of the liver.

While scientists are trying to fit all these pieces of the puzzle together, about a quarter of a million people die in the United Kingdom every year from various forms of cancer. As already emphasized, the majority can be cured if diagnosed early enough and it is crucially important to know what changes in your body you should take seriously and report immediately to your doctor. You will find a list below. Do not panic if you notice any of the following signs. Very often the explanation for your symptoms may be simple and the cause quite benign, but do go to your doctor soon and ask for his advice.

The International Union Against Cancer provides eight warning signs:

1 Lump in the breast, neck, armpit or elsewhere.

2 Any change in a mole or wart be it size or colour.

3 Unexplained weight loss.

4 Chronic indigestion or difficulty in swallowing.

5 Any unexplained change in bowel or bladder habits.

6 Chronic persistent cough or hoarseness.

7 Any sore or ulcer which does not heal.

8 Unusual bleeding or discharge.

Breast cancer

Warning signs:

1 Alteration in the shape of the breast.

2 An unusual lump in the breast.

3 A blood-stained discharge from the nipple.

4 A swelling in the armpit.

There are two very reassuring facts about breast cancer. The first is that the majority of lumps in the breast are not malignant. The second is that early treatment of breast cancer can bring about a complete cure. So seek advice early if you are worried about anything.

There seems to be a genetic factor in the development of breast cancer. The women most at risk are those who have a relative who has had the disease. Other women who have a greater risk than the average population are women with no children, or only one child, women who had their first child after thirty-five, women who have had a number of benign lumps in the breast and women with a late menopause – periods going on after they are fifty-one years old.

Because cancer of the breast is so eminently treatable if discovered early, it is important to know how to perform your own breast examination. You are looking for two main things: *a change in the size, shape or colour of the nipple;* and *a dimpling of the skin over the surface of a lump.*

1 Sit naked in front of a mirror and observe your breasts carefully.

2 Raise your arms above your head to make dimpling of the skin more obvious.

3 Lie down.

4 Feel your breasts with your hand flat and fingers straight.

5 Examine your left breast with your right hand with your left arm stretched back beyond your head.

6 Repeat for your right breast, pressing your fingers gently on to each quarter of the breast.

7 Sit up.

8 Feel in your armpits for any hard lumps (swollen glands).

9 Examine yourself at least once a month in this way and if you detect anything wrong see your doctor within twenty-four hours.

Skin cancer

Warning signs:

1 Moles or birthmarks which begin to grow, bleed, change colour or become tender.

2 An ulcer which does not heal.

3 Any lump in the skin which grows larger.

It is known that skin tumours occur most often in those with skin exposed to too much sun and in fair-skinned people. Most skin tumours however can be easily dealt with and cause very little trouble.

A rodent ulcer is the commonest form of skin tumour and the incidence increases as we get older. It is very common on the face. It starts as a small raised lump whose centre ulcerates as the edges grow outwards and have a rather rolled, curly edge. These tumours are very easily treated with X-rays. The most dangerous skin tumours are those which are brown or black in colour, melanomas, and are growing rapidly in size or becoming inflamed. Radical treatment with excision of surrounding tissue if performed early can have good results.

Cancer of the oesophagus (gullet) and stomach

Warning signs:

1 Any new symptom in the middle-aged person referable to the stomach, e.g. indigestion, vomiting.

2 Persistent indigestion or difficulty in swallowing.

3 Loss of appetite.

4 Stomach pains and vomiting.

5 The appearance of black, tarry stools (due to blood lost in the stomach which changes colour during its passage through the bowel from red to black).

These cancers can be detected very easily by a series of hospital tests which have reached a high degree of technical reliability. Such tests would include a barium meal and gastroscopy (looking at the lining of the stomach through a tube which is swallowed). Stomach cancers are usually treated by surgery and it is possible to eat almost normally even after quite large parts of the stomach have been removed.

Cancer of the lower bowel and rectum

Warning signs:

1 Any unexplained change in bowel habit.
2 The sudden appearance of constipation or diarrhoea.
3 The stool becomes thin and pipe-like.
4 Pain in the bowel.
5 Blood, or pus, or a lot of mucus in the stools.

The results of early treatment by surgery are extremely good and therefore it is important that an early diagnosis is made. Recent theories on the causation of cancers of the bowel are being linked with a diet too rich in fat and low in fibre.

Lung cancer

Warning signs:

1 Chronic persistent cough.
2 Blood in the sputum.
3 Severe pain in the chest.
4 Lingering chest infections.

Other than regular chest X-rays, a method for detecting lung cancer early has not been devised. The chances of recovery are very poor unless diagnosed early, so the only line to follow is prevention.

The question of smoking and lung cancer cannot be avoided. The connection was first raised in 1939 but it is only in the last ten to fifteen years that the relationship between smoking and lung cancer has been examined scientifically and subjected to statistical analysis. For most doctors this association has been shown to be highly significant. This means that the increased chance of developing lung cancer in smokers is not due to coincidence but is directly related to the smoking of cigarettes.

Lung cancer was a rare disease until cigarette smoking became commonplace; now it is one of the commonest forms of cancer. Smokers, regardless of sex, are more likely to develop lung cancer than non-smokers. The risk of cancer increases directly in proportion to the number of cigarettes smoked a day; giving up smoking results in a corresponding reduction in risk. At one time lung cancer was much more common in men than in women and this was reflected in smoking habits. Now that more and more women are smoking the difference between the sexes is narrowing.

Scientists believe that the change from a normal cell to a cancerous cell involves the passage of time and several separate steps. The initial stimulus causes changes in the enzymes in the very nucleus of a cell and causes it to multiply. At this stage the cell is not cancerous but if the changes continue it will become so. It follows that if the initial stimulus is removed at an early stage the multiplying process can be blocked and this has been experimentally demonstrated. This theory fits in very nicely with the observed facts about cigarette smokers who, if they are able to give up smoking, can reduce the risk of developing lung cancer. (For tips on how to control your smoking see p. 77.)

Cancer of the womb and cervix (the neck of the womb)

Warning signs

1 Bleeding after intercourse.

2 Irregular bleeding between periods.

3 Heavy periods, or prolonged bleeding after the period.

Statistically there are certain women who are at greater risk from cancer of the cervix. These are women who have had children, women who have had several partners and women with low incomes. As cancer of the cervix can now be easily diagnosed by a cervical smear every woman should go for a smear test once a year. Cervical cancer found in its early stages can be prevented from spreading by a very simple operation. Cancer of the womb is detected by taking a scraping from the lining and it can also be treated very successfully by surgery if detected early enough.

Cancer of the prostate

Warning signs:

1 Having to get up in the night to pass urine and then only a small quantity.

2 Having to pass urine more frequently.

3 A feeling of urgency to pass urine.

4 Difficulty or discomfort in passing urine.

5 Stools become thin and pipe-like.

Benign prostatic enlargement is very common and causes exactly the same symptoms as a malignant tumour. So while there is probably no need to worry should you develop any of the above symptoms, you should go along to your doctor for an examination and advice. New surgical procedures for removal of the prostate gland, which is found at the base of the bladder in close proximity to the rectum, result in high cure rates.

Today, medicines are available which can cure most forms of early cancer. The majority of doctors believe that improvement in cancer cure rates could be dramatic if more patients went to their doctor sooner. In this context fatal cancer becomes a *preventable* disease.

Some case histories

CANCER OF THE BOWEL Mr F., aged fifty-seven, had always kept a regular daily bowel action without the aid of purgatives and was quick to notice when a day was missed. A few days later he noticed slime and a trace of blood in his motions so he went immediately to his doctor. By jogging his memory, Mr F.'s doctor discovered that for the past month or so the stool had been thinner than before. When he examined Mr F. rectally, he told Mr. F he could feel a slightly hard roughened ring at the top of his rectum, and said he would get Mr F. an appointment to see a specialist as soon as possible.

In the hospital clinic the specialist examined Mr F.'s rectum with a lighted tube so that he could see the constriction and requested Mr F. to come on to his ward for further tests. A week later, Mr F. was admitted and had a barium enema the next day. The following evening the specialist told Mr F. and his wife that he thought Mr F. had an early cancer of the rectum and he would like to operate. The operation would involve cutting out the growth and a portion of bowel, sewing up the rectum and bringing the bowel to open on to the abdominal wall in the form of a colostomy. The surgeon explained how a colostomy worked, answered Mr and Mrs F.'s questions and said he would give them twenty-four hours to think it over. With the operation he gave Mr F. a seventy per cent chance of being fit and well in five years. Without it, but with X-ray therapy, he gave him a ten per cent chance of being alive in five years.

Mr and Mrs F. decided in favour of surgery and the difficult four-hour-long operation was a success. Two days after the operation Mr F.'s abdomen became swollen with gas and it was diagnosed that his bowel was paralyzed* as a result of the operation. He was fed intravenously, while all fluid was withdrawn from his

* Post-operative paralysis of the bowel: This condition is called paralytic ileus and is a not infrequent consequence of any operation which involves handling the intestines. It is a sort of state of shock of the bowel which invariably recovers if treated with a 'drip and suck' routine. It is certainly not a reflection of the surgeon's skill, but the result of the mechanical intervention that is necessary for abdominal operations.

stomach via a tube passed through his nose. This treatment went well; within a few days he was taking liquids and a week later he was eating a semi-solid diet. His colostomy was working well too, if slightly more often than he was used to, and he was becoming accustomed to wearing and changing the colostomy bags and the hygiene routine for cleaning and looking after the skin. He did not mind the bland food though he missed onions which were a great favourite with him, and quickly learned to restrict himself to the items on his specially designed diet which kept his bowel fairly quiet.

Mr F. has had his colostomy for several years now. Not even his wife can detect any smell and, since he generally wears loose-fitting sweaters, none but Mr F.'s closest friends are aware of his colostomy. Mr F. is active and has never been fitter and he and his wife wouldn't miss their summer holiday abroad for anything.

CANCER OF THE LUNG Eighteen months ago Mr B., aged sixty-two, noticed the odd speck of blood in his sputum for about two or three days and then it disappeared. It reappeared ten days later and persisted so he went to his doctor.

He had smoked about thirty-five untipped cigarettes a day since he joined the navy as a lad of sixteen and always had a cough in the morning. He had not noticed any shortness of breath nor had he experienced any pains in his chest, but over the past six to nine months felt that he had lost some weight because his trousers had got slack around his waist. His doctor put him on the scales and to Mr B.'s astonishment he found he was 20 lb lighter than he had been when he had had a medical two years before.

His doctor listened to his chest and suggested he had an X-ray and that he should come back to see him in a week when he would have the report. The report described a large shadow in the right lung with evidence of spread. The picture pointed to a fairly advanced and rapidly growing cancer. Mr B. was referred immediately to see a surgeon who explained that he had lung cancer and told him the preferred method of treatment was with powerful anti-cancer drugs. In collaboration with a colleague he gave Mr B. several courses of this therapy. X-rays showed that the tumour was shrinking. Mr B.'s appetite picked up and he put on a little weight. He returned every three months for hospital check-ups and remained well. He continued to smoke.

A year ago, Mr B. noticed that his abdomen was becoming swollen and he had a dragging feeling in his left side. When his doctor examined him he found that his liver was enlarged, and he sent Mr B. immediately to see his surgeon who admitted him to hospital for investigation. Tests revealed that the lung cancer had spread to Mr B.'s liver and further courses of anti-cancer drugs were prescribed, this time given into a vein in Mr B.'s arm. On this occasion the powerful drugs affected his blood making him anaemic and Mr B. had to have two blood transfusions. He remained weak and his appetite was poor, but after three weeks in hospital he was well enough to return home to convalesce.

Five months ago Mr B. started to go downhill rapidly and had to be confined to bed. He began to have severe headaches which required strong pain-killers to relieve them. He could eat very little and became extremely thin.

Three weeks ago Mr B. passed into a coma and was readmitted to hospital. He was fed through a drip into his arm but he never regained consciousness and died two weeks after admission.

Postmortem revealed a large, highly malignant tumour which had invaded most of the right lung, advanced secondary deposits in the liver and fairly recent secondaries in the brain.

BREAST CANCER Mrs W., aged thirty-three years, married and childless, noticed a small hard pea-shaped lump in the upper outer quarter of her right breast. As her breasts became nodular to the touch with the approach of each period, she thought nothing of it. Three days later she felt it again and told her husband about it. He insisted she saw the doctor and she made an appointment to see her GP the next day. Her doctor examined the lump and said although he did not think it would be anything serious he wanted her seen quickly by a surgeon in case it was. Mrs W. was able to see a specialist the following day (as can anyone with any of the symptoms described on p. 92). He told her it was his standard practice to operate as quickly as possible. As she had come to him soon after discovering the lump and as he had found no swollen glands in her armpit, he would remove only the lump (lumpectomy) and not the breast (mastectomy)*. He would have the lump examined and if it proved to be malignant† he would remove some of the glands from the armpit to look for spread of the tumour.

Mrs W. was admitted to hospital forty-eight hours later and went to surgery the following morning. When she awoke she had a drain in the wound which was connected to a bottle which she had to carry around with her wherever she went. Her breast was intact. The day after the operation her surgeon came to see her and told her the lump was cancer and it was a very malignant type so while all the glands he had removed were found to be free of tumour, he still wanted her to have post-operative X-ray therapy to kill off any remaining tumour cells.

Five days later the stitches were removed from the wound and Mrs W. returned home. During the following weeks she attended the out-patient

* Removal of the tumour: Opinions vary as to how the tumour should be removed, from the simplest operation for early tumours, lumpectomy, to the most radical, total mastectomy for tumours which have progressed, and which involves removal of the glands of the armpit.

† Nature of the tumour: Mrs W.'s surgeon discussed openly with her the possible malignant nature of the lump in her breast. If you ask your surgeon to be frank with you he will do the same.

radiography department for X-ray therapy. After the first session she felt weak, giddy and sick* and went back to her GP. He told her that her symptoms were probably due to worry and gave her a tranquillizer to help her over the understandable anxiety. She took them only for two weeks then stopped them because she felt she could cope and the symptoms had not returned.

It is now three and a half years since her operation. Mrs W. attends out-patients for check-ups every six months. On her last visit two months ago, she was told all was well. She is fit and healthy and hardly ever thinks about the fact that she *had* breast cancer.

* Symptoms after radiotherapy: Mrs W. was having fairly light doses of X-ray therapy because she has a fair skin and it was important not to burn it, so her sensations of sickness, dizziness and weakness were most probably psychosomatic. These symptoms, however, quite frequently accompany *deep* X-ray therapy.

8 How Not to Mistreat Your Body

Smoking

Smoking is one of the most serious ways in which we mistreat our bodies. Its damaging and frequently life-destroying properties are discussed in detail in three other chapters: on pp. 94–5 in 'Cancer'; on p. 69 in 'How to Keep a Healthy Heart'; and on pp. 75–7 in 'Having a Healthy Chest'. Advice on how to control your smoking can be found on p. 77.

It is worth remembering that even smokers who are otherwise quite healthy are suffering without knowing it. Cigarette smoke in the lungs interferes with the oxygenation of the blood and the haemoglobin, the pigment in the red blood cells that carries oxygen around the body, is rendered useless for oxygen transport by being changed to methaemaglobin.

Travel and jet-lag

Ten years ago I flew to San Francisco and the following day attended a rather high-powered scientific meeting where I was called upon to participate. To my horror I found that I not only failed to remember facts with which I was entirely conversant, but worse, I could not find the words to express myself. I thought I was cracking up. Without knowing it, I was suffering from what we now know as jet-lag. It was a full four years later, when I was one of the medical team who conducted a detailed experiment to examine the effects of jet-lag, that I discovered what I had experienced a few years earlier was absolutely classical of the jet-lag syndrome.

Jet-lag can show itself in any of the following:

1 Inability to remember well-known facts.
2 Inability to find technical words with which one is ordinarily familiar.
3 Inability to make decisions.
4 Inability to take into account several different aspects of a problem to form a solution.
5 Inability to stay awake in the middle of the day.
6 Inability to go to sleep in the middle of the night.
7 Waking in the small hours of the morning.

8 Lack of desire to eat at prescribed times.
9 Attacks of nausea, dizziness.
10 Inability to concentrate.
11 Inattention to detail.
12 Slow reflex actions.
13 Decrease in the powers of judgement.

It can be seen that one's intellectual powers are seriously affected when one is suffering from jet-lag. This has enormous implications to itinerant politicians or senior business executives who are expected not only to attend high-level business meetings but to make decisions with important consequences while suffering from jet-lag.

While many *simulated* experiments have been carried out to examine the effect of jet-lag, an almost definitive 'real situation' experiment was done with fourteen volunteers who were flown from London to the west coast of America and back again. Everyone was subjected to four-hourly testing for the whole four weeks of the study. The sort of tests we performed were: psychological (tests on the heart, e.g. electrocardiographic examination, blood-pressure); biochemical (e.g. blood and urine hormone levels); intellectual (tests of decision making, tests of accuracy, tests of attention to detail); physiological (tests of mood change, tests of ability to cope with problems); sleep (electro-encephalographic examination of sleep patterns in a sleep laboratory by recording brain-waves all through the night). At the end of the study we had shown that every test we performed was affected by jet-lag – all the tests were in the abnormal range. What is more, we showed that for journeys westward, i.e. London to Los Angeles, it took seven to nine days for the tests to return to normal levels, and for journeys eastward, i.e. Los Angeles to London, it took more than eleven days, which was the longest time we were able to hold our subjects captive after their return to the United Kingdom.

The journey from London to the west coast of America involves a time-change of eight or nine hours, according to whether or not we are on summer time. The journey to New York involves a time-change of five or six hours. As a rough guide it takes the body one day to adjust for each hour of time-change. So it takes roughly five to six days after you arrive in New York for your body to have caught up with New York time.

Though we do not know the precise cause of jet-lag we do know that in broad terms it is due to a disturbance of our biological rhythms. Nearly every important function within our body, including waking, sleeping, eating, peaks of intellectual activity, etc. are controlled by internal biological clocks. When we travel to a far distant place we find that our internal clock is, say, at midnight, but the societal clock around us is at 6 a.m.; our bodies are called upon to do things at 6 a.m. which they would not normally do for another six hours. This throws out the timing of all our internal rhythms and until they can fit themselves, or lock-on, to the societal rhythm around us, we do not behave or work normally.

Is there anything we can do to help our bodies adjust to this trauma? Yes, there is. If we have to attend an important meeting in a foreign land, which involves a time-zone change, we should try to organize our schedule so that we arrive there a day or two early to allow some adjustment to the societal time before going into our meetings.

Although hardened jet travellers are always prepared to give you their particular recipe for dealing with jet-lag, there seem to be two generally accepted ways of adjusting. One school of thought says that as soon as you arrive you should 'lock-on' to societal time and do whatever the people around you are doing regardless of what time it is in your own day. And whilst sleep deprivation *per se* has very little to do with jet-lag, the second school of thought says that a good long sleep as soon as you have made a time-zone change is the key to getting back to normal fast. It is advocated that you take sleeping pills to get this sleep if it does not come naturally.

Sun worship

Being of a dermatological bent, I can never understand why so many people chase the sun and the suntan that goes with it rather than staying pale and interesting. We all need some sun of course, because vitamin D is manufactured in the skin from an inactive substance and is activated by sunlight. We get enough sunshine, however, from the sun that reaches our skin during our normal daily life to ensure that we have plenty of vitamin D; there is no need to strip to get it.

All dermatologists know that the sun's rays are harmful and destructive to the skin. Many years ago a professor of dermatology did a beautiful experiment which shows just how destructive the ultraviolet rays in sunlight are to skin. He took small pieces of skin from the back of a baby's hand, from the baby's bottom, from the back of the hand of an octogenarian, and from his bottom, and compared their appearance under a microscope. What he found was this: the skin from the baby's bottom, the back of the baby's hand and from the eighty-year-old's bottom were identical in appearance, whereas the skin from the back of the old man's hand was showing all the classical destructive changes of ageing. Virtually the only difference between this particular specimen and the other three was the fact that it had been exposed to sunlight for eighty years.

There are two main changes that ultraviolet radiation produces in the skin. One is ageing, the other is to increase the tendency to develop cancer of the skin.

When the skin ages it loses its suppleness, its soft pliant quality and its plumpness. It becomes thin, it sags, it is inelastic and it wrinkles. One of the major factors involved in this deterioration is a change deep in the dermis of the skin which involves collagen.

Collagen is a complex protein which lies in bundles that, in youth, are arranged in beautiful parallel layers. These bundles contract and relax and give the skin pliancy and suppleness and the ability to spring back into shape when distorted. As we age, the collagen bundles begin to disintegrate and break up. This process gradually undermines the suppleness of the skin and as time progresses, results in the appearance of wrinkles and crow's feet. The effect of ultraviolet radiation on collagen is exactly the same as ageing, and chronic prolonged exposure to sunlight will produce disruption of collagen and premature ageing of the skin. So if you want wrinkles when you are thirty, the way to do it is to sit out in the sun whenever you can.

The process whereby the skin tans is simply the skin's response to injury. Ultraviolet light, if it penetrates through the upper layers of the skin into the deeper layers, leaves a trail of damaged tissue. We have a natural sunscreen in our skin called melanin and people living in parts of the world where there are many hours of sunshine have darker skin than those who live where the number of sunshine hours is low. Hence we have shades of skin all the way down from black to white. When pale-skinned people are exposed to bright sunlight for many hours a day the skin starts to produce more melanin to screen off the harmful elements of the sun's rays to protect itself. The more we expose ourselves to sunlight the more melanin is produced. We all have the same number of melanin cells but the darker the skin the more melanin the cells can produce.

The initial response to sunlight, however, may be inflammation, with all the signs of sunburn and possibly even the dangerous condition of sunstroke, where the skin becomes so inflamed that it cannot perform its function of regulating the body's temperature. A person with sunstroke is very ill indeed, with a high temperature which is difficult to bring down. After several days in bright strong sunshine the skin reaches a happy balance with its environment and is producing melanin at a sufficiently high rate to screen off the dangerous elements of sunlight. At this point our skins are deeply tanned.

The other harmful aspect of sunlight is its propensity to produce malignant change in the skin. In most people the tendency of the skin to produce malignant tumours is directly proportional to the number of sunlight hours it is exposed to. If you live in a country like Australia or South Africa where the average number of sunlight hours per day for every day of the year is approaching ten, then you will be exposed to more sunlight hours in fewer years than you will if you live in a country like sun-starved England. So whereas in Australia it may take ten or fifteen years to be exposed to the number of sunlight hours which will stimulate a malignant change in skin growth, in England it may take twenty-five to thirty. Evidence of this connection is the relatively high incidence of skin cancer in countries where there is a lot of sunshine compared to the incidence where there is little. Of course all of us have accumulated many hours of exposure to sunlight as we approach old age in those parts of the body which are habitually exposed to the sun. Hence the incidence of skin malignancy on the back of the hands and face is higher than in those parts of the skin which are kept covered.

If you must go out in the sun wear a shady hat to protect the delicate skin of your face, use lots of moisturizer (three or four times a day) and a sun-screen cream. Wear sun-glasses in glaring sun, especially in snow or if you are reading. If you must be brown, better get it out of a bottle.

Posture

When we ceased to be quadrupeds and began to walk around on two legs, the spinal column had to cope with the engineering stress of swinging through 90° and transmitting the weight of our head and shoulders down through our hip-joints, legs and knees to our feet. In doing so it took up several curvatures.

It is only in the very young, however, that you will see these healthy curves still intact. Young children with actively exercised muscles and supple joints naturally hold themselves in the position where their spine can function optimally. It so happens that this position is the one which is best for good breathing, good digestion, good cardiac function, and which puts the least strain on all the other joints, muscles and nerves of the back, shoulders, hips and limbs.

As we get older our joints stiffen, our muscles become unfit and we tend to slouch. Injury may make us hold ourselves in a special way to protect an injured part and so put an extra stress on a corresponding part. Some people place a strain on their natural posture because they are in a profession which demands it; for example, models, who traditionally pose with one hip thrown forward. A very famous model had such a misshapen pelvis from constantly having to take up the hand on hip, hip pushed sideways stance, that she was unable to have babies normally and had to have children by Caesarean section. For all these reasons the curvature of our spine tends to flatten out as we get older, leading to many of the aches and pains in the back that are a familiar part of ageing.

The spine takes a tremendous amount of wear and tear just in our normal everyday life. Think of the movement that occurs at the neck as we move our head from side to side and up and down, simply in looking at things. Because of its crucial position in the body, the spine is subjected to strains all of the day and

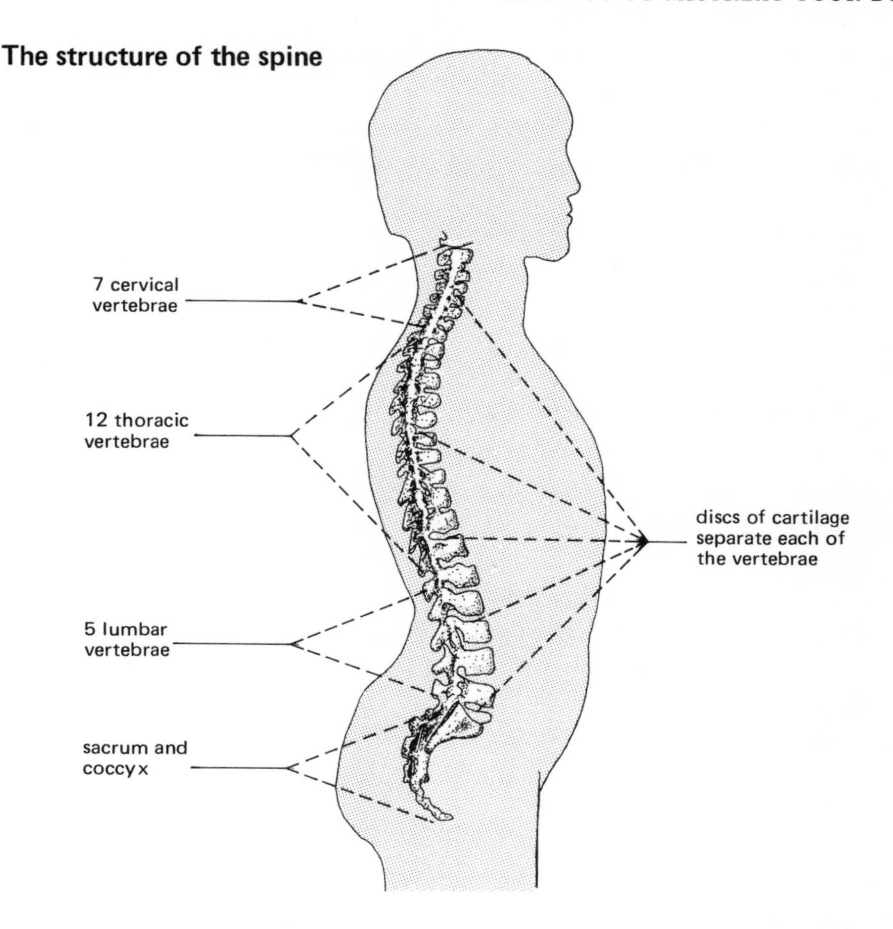

most of the night too if we do not sleep on a mattress which supports the back. Think of the stresses on the lower part of the back because of the bending, stooping, twisting, turning that we have to do in the course of a normal day. An artificial joint would wear out in a very short time given this amount of stress, so it is not surprising that our spinal joints tend to wear out too. If we stand or sit, lift or bend wrongly, if we walk incorrectly, if we drive in a bumpy car, we are overworking our spine and its muscles and ligaments. Even if we do not injure them, we overtire them and that tiredness can lead to backache as opposed to back pain.

The statistics on back pain are pretty staggering: four out of five people will have back pain at some time in their lives; every day at least one in five of the adult population will suffer agonizing back pain; about 56,000 people will be unable to go to work every day because of back pain; a few people will face a lifetime of very severe pain which may affect their jobs, their family and their emotional lives; back pain costs more than £300 million each year in terms of medical care, sickness benefits and lost production.

Because the lower back is pivotal in all the movements of the body, once it has been injured it very rarely returns to normal. No matter how much care is taken to make sure that the injury is healed, there is always a certain weakness left. It is therefore very important to learn how to use your back properly, to strain it as little as possible to prevent injury from ever occurring.

There are proper ways to stand, sit, bend, lift and walk which throw the strain of all these movements on to much stronger muscles and joints than the spine – joints which are more stable and less likely to be injured; joints which are not cushioned by the inter-vertebral discs that can be injured so easily, take so long to heal and cause so much pain during the healing process. So it is just commonsense to use the stronger muscles and joints to do the work of the spine and to protect it from being overstrained.

To assume good posture when standing, hold your shoulders firmly, but not rigidly, back and down, with your head up and your tummy pulled in. There is nothing sergeant-major-like about this. If you fix your arms to your sides and your shoulders back too rigidly you will find that your breathing is restricted. Just taking up this posture helps to accentuate the curvatures of the spine and to keep it well supported by the muscles of the back and shoulders.

Both in our jobs and at home we spend much of our time sitting so we should make sure that we are sitting in well-designed chairs. The feature of a chair

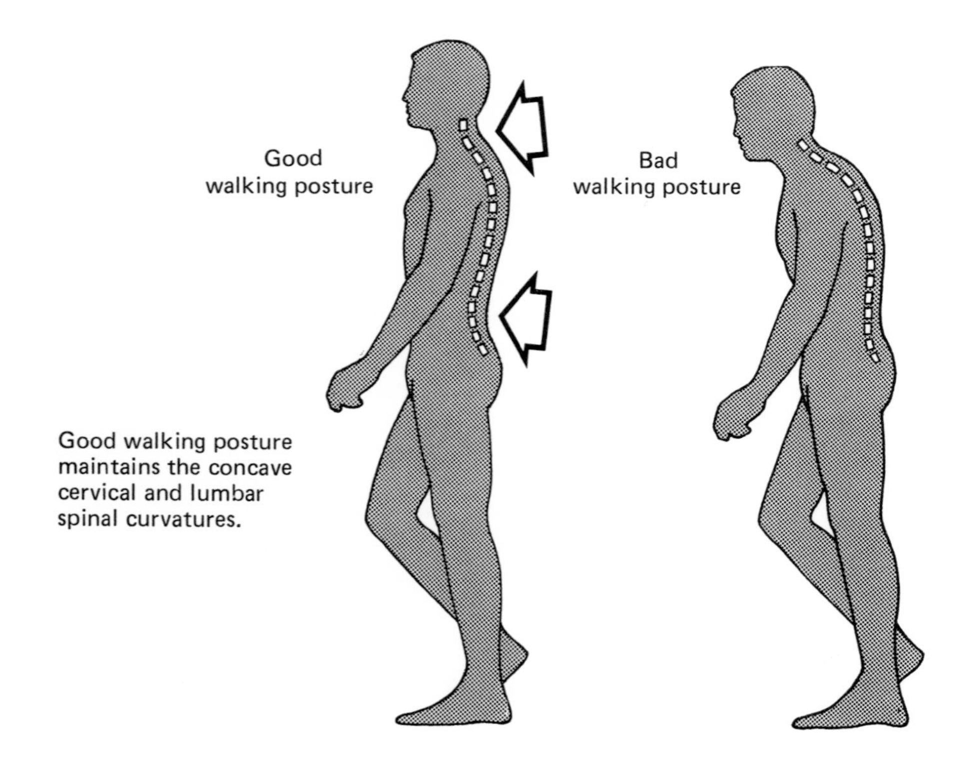

Good walking posture maintains the concave cervical and lumbar spinal curvatures.

which is good for posture is one which keeps the angle of the spine to the hip at about 120° ensuring maximum comfort and minimum strain on spinal joints and spinal muscles. In addition, a well-designed chair should be convex where the back joins the seat so that the lower part of our spine is well supported. Look out for this feature when you are buying new chairs and when buying a car.

We spend a great deal of time driving and it is essential both for driving

Make sure the car seat supports you correctly when driving.

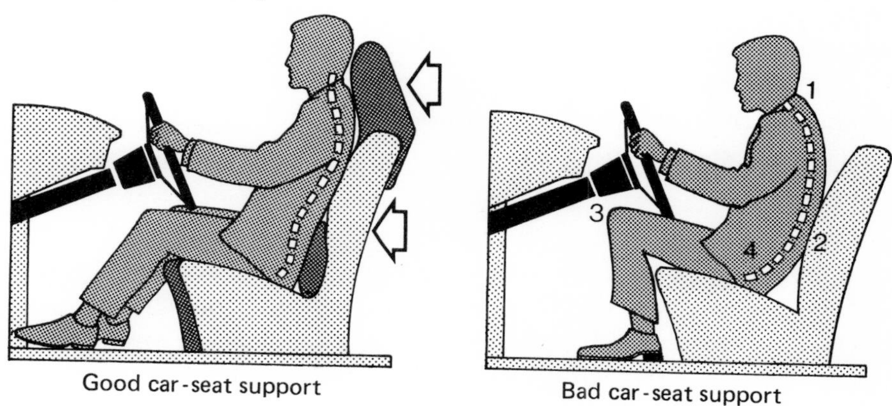

Good car-seat support

Bad car-seat support

In a badly-designed car seat or when sitting in an incorrect driving position:

1 The shoulders slump and the cervical spine curves convexly.
2 The lumbar curvature is lost and becomes convex.
3 The knees are allowed to bend and increase the hip angle beyond the desired 120° (4).

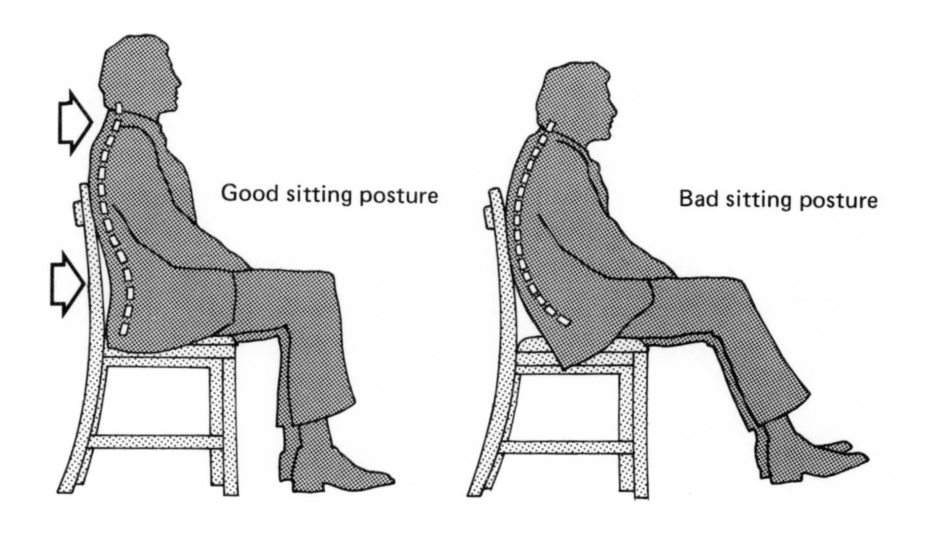

comfort and safety that our car seats are designed to support the lower part of the spine. If you have a car in which the seats do not provide this support, most car accessory shops can provide you with a cushion which you can fit into the lower part of your seat.

Considering that we spend approximately one-third of our lives asleep, it is worth paying some attention to the sort of mattresses we sleep on. While most of us love fluffy, downy, soft mattresses, they are extremely bad for our backs since they allow the spine to curve outwards. A firm mattress is much better than a soft one. Old-fashioned beds with a box which provides an inflexible base are better than those without. Most of us know someone who, having injured his back, is told by their doctor that the best way of curing back pain is to put an old door underneath the mattress to support the back during the night. What is good when we are in pain is even better when we are not, because it is preventing an overworked spine from being strained.

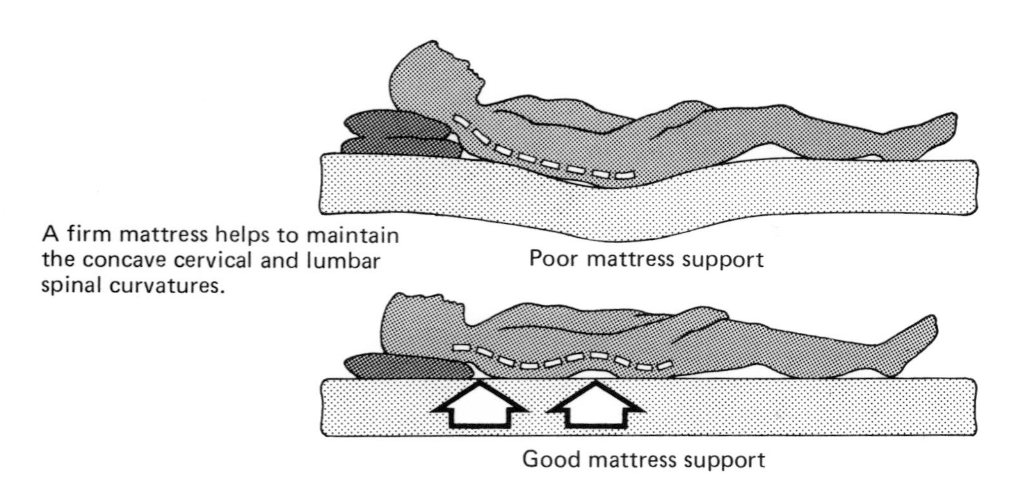

A firm mattress helps to maintain the concave cervical and lumbar spinal curvatures.

Many back injuries occur when simple everyday tasks are attempted in the wrong way, or when you try to do something very strenuously when you are unfit. The booklet, *Avoiding Back Trouble*, published by the Consumers' Association, gives some very useful tips on how to avoid injuring your back and describes in detail how you should cope with everyday household tasks in the most efficient way; these include bed-making, bathing the baby, cleaning the floor, the bath and the windows, jobs in the kitchen, washing your hair, shaving, washing and ironing, moving furniture, carrying luggage and moving an invalid or an unconscious person. The booklet also gives tips on how to stand properly and how to lift heavy objects correctly. To anyone who now has or has had an injury to their back, I would recommend this booklet highly. (See also **Back pain**, p. 143.)

Alcohol

Alcohol, unlike smoking, is not always bad for you; a little can even be beneficial. But the majority of us over-indulge sometimes and that hangover feeling is really a very good index to how much we are punishing our bodies. When drinking a little becomes drinking a lot, it ceases to be a pleasure; it soon becomes a dangerous addiction which can lead to disease and even death. Furthermore, while alcoholism is a self-inflicted illness, its effects go beyond individual drinkers. It can result in the break-up of marriages, the alienation of one's children, dismissal from a job, and in fatal injuries to others.

It is thought that as many as half a million people in England and Wales alone have a serious drinking problem and the proportion is even higher in Scotland. Between 1959 and 1973 admissions to hospital for the treatment of alcoholism rose by more than five hundred per cent and if the trend continues, in ten years' time alcoholism will account for about a quarter of all admissions to psychiatric hospitals. In parallel with this increasing intake of alcohol are criminal convictions for alcohol-related offences.

The physical effects of alcoholism are awful. About two-thirds of chronic alcoholics suffer from a condition of the liver called fatty infiltration, and about ten in every hundred from cirrhosis of the liver. The death rate from cirrhosis of the liver went up by about thirty per cent between 1963 and 1973. The nervous damage that can be caused by alcohol is extensive and disabling. The earliest changes involve the nerves in the hands and the feet and is called polyneuritis. It causes tingling in the fingers and toes and cramps in the legs. The ability to judge distances quite often fails, as does the co-ordination of hand and foot and eye. And then in later stages, the memory goes and brain damage can be permanent. Quite a number of alcoholics suffer from peptic ulcers, but it is not known if this results directly from the intake of alcohol.

Like any drug that can make you feel good, alcohol is potentially addictive. What can start as social drinking can progress to taking a drink for the relief of a problem, nervousness, or anxiety, to habitual social drinking and taking a drink every time you become stressed. If this is not checked you can then go on into the risky phase which is only a step away from the critical phase. The risky phase shows itself because one becomes increasingly tolerant of alcohol and needs to take more and more to achieve the desired effect. Also you begin to drink surreptitiously which is when dependence on alcohol really begins to show itself. You have entered the critical phase when you are unable to stop drinking and find yourself breaking promises and resolutions to stop drinking, avoiding family and friends, and neglecting food. This goes on to having to take an early morning drink in order to start the day and having to keep on drinking to get through it.

We can help ourselves to avoid the slippery slope to alcoholism by drinking healthily. We should be good hosts and offer our friends more non-alcoholic drinks. Try to drink an equal quantity of water with your alcohol. Try to eat a snack while you drink. Cut down on the aperitifs and on the liqueurs. Be prepared for a few snide comments from your friends, and miss out on a round in the pub or order a half pint when you would ordinarily order a pint, or even a non-alcoholic drink.

If you do take more alcohol than is good for you, you are probably neglecting your diet. The most important precaution you must take is to make sure you get plenty of vitamins, especially the B vitamins. Most alcoholics suffer from vitamin B deficiency which affects the nerves, the first signs being pins and needles in the hands and feet. (For foods which are good sources of vitamin B, see p. 42.)

We can also help our children by maintaining a sensible attitude to drinking in the home. We know, for instance, that there is a higher incidence of alcoholism in the children of alcoholics, so the very fact that you are not an alcoholic yourself is doing a service to your children. So, as with many other pleasures in life, try to teach your children discrimination and to take everything in moderation.

You can also do your baby a service before it is born by not drinking heavily in pregnancy. A mother who drinks heavily puts her baby at risk. A professor in Germany has estimated that one in three alcoholic mothers will probably have a handicapped child. We owe it to our babies not to allow this to happen.

Sleep

From the baby who sleep fifteen hours out of twenty-four to the seventy-year-old who naps for only four, we all need sleep. To ignore the need can have unpleasant consequences, even if it is just the knowledge that we are functioning at less than our best. For some, chronic lack of sleep can lead to a complete emotional breakdown. The fact that sleep deprivation is used as a method of breaking an individual's will is good evidence that we need a proper night's sleep.

Why do our bodies *need* sleep? To a certain extent we are not in control of our need because the act of going to sleep may be chemically or hormonally engineered. Our bodies have an innate twenty-four-hour rhythm imposed upon them, which involves the outpouring of certain hormones at certain times of the day and night. One hormone, cortisol, is turned on at about 4–5 a.m. and initiates our arousal from sleep. From about 8 p.m. onwards the level of cortisol falls off; by midnight it is very low and it is mainly responsible for the fact that we feel sleepy at night time.

Sleep is so important that the brain has built at least two centres connected with sleep; one sends us off to sleep, the other keeps us asleep. The first one, which makes us drop off, is activated by such cues as darkness, habit, seeing other people going to sleep, physical tiredness and intellectual fatigue. The second one is probably triggered by chemical changes in brain cells.

One descriptive analogy of the need to sleep is the need for a spent battery to recharge itself and it is an easy matter to imagine the body recovering from the day's activities by sleeping. For the average human being sixteen or seventeen hours of wakefulness create the need to recharge. There is some physiological research in support of the 'recharge' theory. Brain cells can only function when they contain what appear under the microscope to be granules. When one feels in need of sleep brain cells are almost completely devoid of granules. After several hours of sleep they are replenished. It is not just the brain that is recharging itself during sleep, other organs are too. The whole body goes into a state of semi-hibernation – we breathe slowly, and breathing is usually shallow; the heart-rate drops as does the body temperature; digestion virtually ceases and so does the formation of urine.

But for me the most attractive theory about the need to sleep is that *we sleep to dream.* Here again there is a technological analogy which gives the theory credence. The brain has been likened to a computer, a computer which is absorbing more information than any electronic equivalent. But the most complex computer will blow a fuse if every now and then the circuits aren't cleared of redundant information. Many sleep scientists believe that during dreams – which occur several times whenever we sleep – our computer, the brain, clears its circuits.

The most recent theory of dreams postulates that it is only during dreams that we can manufacture certain chemicals that are needed for proper intellectual functioning. If we sleep, but don't dream, because we are prevented from doing so by drugs or are wakened during dreaming, these essential chemicals cannot be manufactured. Some sleeping pills, e.g. barbiturates, induce sleep but prevent dreaming and this is thought to be why they are also followed by a hangover feeling in the morning. Alcohol induced sleep is unsatisfactory for a similar reason. The most modern hypnotics hardly interfere with dreaming at all and give good quality sleep.

Dreaming is accompanied by a change in brain-wave activity. In sleep laboratories, dreaming activity has been followed on electro-encephalographic recordings. If you allow volunteers to sleep and wake them every time dreaming starts, they exhibit all the symptoms of profound sleep deprivation.

Whether or not you believe Winston Churchill who said: 'A man needs six hours sleep, a boy needs seven, and only women and fools need more,' make sure you get your quota if you wish to keep your mind and your body in tip-top condition. (See also **Insomnia**, pp. 177–8.)

Irregular eating

Most working adults require two good meals a day. It does not make a lot of difference what time of day you eat, with two exceptions: it is not a good idea to skip breakfast with a full working day ahead of you and lunch four or five hours away; it is not a good idea to have a main meal late at night when your digestive system is closing down for the night and the whole metabolism of the body is shifting into a low gear. In both cases you are making unfair demands on your body which will lower its performance and health.

You will be giving your body a hard time if you treat it to a typical pub lunch as well. A recent experiment performed on volunteer subjects by Professor Vincent Marks of the University of Surrey attracted wide publicity. It examined the effects on the efficiency of the British worker who indulges in a pub lunch. It concluded that a beer and a sandwich, or a gin and tonic and a snack, could be blamed for a lowering of productivity in the afternoon.

Apparently men or women who have a few drinks and a sandwich at lunch time are likely to feel tired, suffer from lack of concentration and an increased tendency to make errors of judgement in the afternoon. By the time they go home they have probably got a headache, and may be feeling irritable and insecure. Work suffers and so does family life.

Professor Marks advances a simple theory to explain these phenomena; the body responds to the high carbohydrate intake of the pub lunch and the resultant soaring blood sugar level by pumping out a huge and sometimes excessive quantity of insulin. The outcome is a rapid clearing of sugar from the blood which may be so efficient that there is a transient phase of hypoglycaemia (too little sugar in the blood). The very low blood sugar levels account for the late afternoon symptoms. So don't punish your body unnecessarily with a drink and some crisps. By all means have a drink, but take sufficient food with it so that the effect of a sudden surge of insulin into the blood is compensated by the continuous absorption of sugar from the digestive tract. That way the notorious post-lunch dip is prevented.

9 The Beauty Game

Like most people I have a basic distrust of over-kill, and I shrink from anything which is being oversold. Consumer advertising is peppered with both, unlike medical advertising which must conform to an enforced ethical code. In consumer advertising, no product carries more appealing messages and promises than the beauty product.

The reality behind beauty advertisements

Every time I see an advertisement for a cosmetic claiming that if I use it for three or four days I shall be able to 'see' and 'feel' the 'difference', I feel angry and insulted, especially if the product makes a claim to remove wrinkles or change the texture of the skin. Nothing applied to the skin can remove wrinkles and nothing applied to the skin can change its texture. Such an advertisement stretches the credibility at the level of basic common sense. But to anyone who knows anything about the physiology of the skin it is an insult. There is no basis yet known to science to justify the claims. Furthermore, it is well nigh impossible to get hold of the evidence on which the claims are based for independent scientific scrutiny.

Beauty advertisements make me angry because they are seducing the public into the purchase of products on the basis of an unproven claim. The seduction often turns out to be an extremely expensive one. That should come as no surprise because the cost of the advertisement must be covered in the price of the product, and the price is further inflated by the cost of the glamorous packaging. In the end, only a fraction of the good money we pay goes on what has been so extravagantly packaged and glossily advertised.

Beauty advertisements make me angry because changing the natural constitution of your skin is no more possible than is changing the colour of your eyes. To all intents and purposes you are bequeathed your skin by your parents. Its quality is genetically determined as are its faults. By far the most important factor in determining a predisposition to acne, wrinkles or any other defect, or the acquisition of an unblemished skin, or one which remains unwrinkled into middle age, or one which looks ten years younger than you do, is *what sort of skin your mother and father had.*

Beauty advertisements make me angry because the physiology of the skin (the way it works) and the anatomy of the skin (its structure) do not permit anything from the outside to affect the health of the skin on the inside. The way the skin looks and feels on the outside can only be changed from the inside. For the skin grows from within outwards, and to affect the health of the skin we must affect the health of the person wearing the skin. The skin is nourished from within, it is fed from within, and the only way that you can change it is by changing it from within.

So even if product X can change the skin in any measurable way it can only change it transiently and this is never stated in the advertisement. And transiently, in terms of the skin, is no more than a few hours. Scientists know of no way in which cosmetics, particularly those containing so-called hormones and collagen, can penetrate to the single layer of living cells deep in the skin and affect them in any way. Collagen, for instance, is too large a molecule to penetrate even the upper layers of the skin. Hormones, by law, cannot be sold over the counter in quantities which are active. In such quantities they must be sold under prescription. It follows that if you can buy a product containing 'hormones' without a prescription it does not have any hormonal effect.

Cosmetic routines

Having understood some of the basic physiology (see p. 40) of the skin we can make certain judgements about cosmetics and the cosmetic routines laid down by beauty experts as though they were written in tablets of stone. Beauty routines, while good in themselves, need not be rigidly adhered to as though they were the *sine qua non* of looking after the skin. While they may have merit, there is no special magic about cleansing, toning and nourishing. Beauticians' programmes are not the be-all and end-all of keeping your skin in good condition. Nor is using expensive products necessarily any better than using cheap ones.

Do, by all means, cleanse your skin, but not necessarily last thing at night and not necessarily with a specially designed cleanser. There is nothing better than a wash with mild baby soap for people who have an oily skin, and for those with drier skins, baby lotion will cleanse, nourish and moisturize your skin if you put it on after you remove your make-up and underneath a new one. There is no law which says you must remove your make-up at night, though some women feel unclean if they do not. On the contrary, it is unphysiological to clean and nourish your skin at night because the skin is virtually dormant in the evening. The skin grows during the early hours of the morning and just after lunch. It would therefore make much more sense to undertake your beauty routine at either or both of these times. Besides, why should your husband be the only man in your life who sees you without any make-up at all?

Moisturizers

I am not a proponent of beauty treatments which have a transient effect on the skin, e.g. face-packs, but I think it is worth making particular mention of moisturizing the skin. Beauticians have a tendency to make this a complicated business but it is very simple. There are only two ways to moisturize the skin: either you can put water into the skin, or you can prevent water being lost from the skin. The first is usually done by applying a cream formulated from oil and water in such a way that the oil can cling to the skin and thereby hold water on its surface. The second is done by applying a more greasy cream similar to the natural sebum produced by sebaceous glands in the skin. This greasy substance forms a film over the skin which prevents water from getting out. The water content in the skin temporarily rises and the skin becomes moisturized.

The second method is by far the more efficient and by far the longer lasting. It is possible to buy fairly inexpensive creams which mimic natural sebum and when applied to the skin will trap moisture for several hours. These latter creams are usually applied under make-up and their barrier effect can last until you remove it. The first type of moisturizer, those that put water into the skin, have a very transient effect. Some of them may last only minutes, rarely longer than a couple of hours. These creams are light and fluffy and when smoothed on the skin give it a soft, pliable feel and disappear in a few minutes.

Hazards of cosmetics

Cost aside, there are good reasons for using simple, pure, inexpensive cosmetics. One is that cosmetics can produce allergies. The more complicated the recipe for any particular cosmetic, the greater the chance of developing an allergy to it and the more difficult to track down the offending substance. A fairly common ingredient of cosmetics is known to be a potent allergen. (A potent allergen causes skin sensitivities and skin allergies in a large number of people.) This is lanolin or wool alcohol which is the base of many creams. A study done at the allergy clinic in St John's Hospital for Skin Diseases in London showed that forty-five per cent of women who come into the clinic with dermatitis are sensitive to lanolin. Many of these allergies are low grade and not easily detected. Some women who are suffering from lanolin allergy may buy more of the cosmetic in the hope that it will make their skin better, whereas it can only make their skin worse.

Allergies to cosmetics are many and varied – as different as allergy to mascara and allergy to nail varnish. These two very different allergies may show themselves in exactly the same way. Puffiness of the eyelids and swelling round the eyes are common expressions of an allergy to mascara and unlikely though it may seem, they are just as frequently seen in patients with an allergy to nail varnish. In nail varnish allergy, rashes and hives (nettle rash) can develop wherever the skin is touched by the polish. You are not always conscious of it but you are constantly putting your fingers to your mouth, nose and eyes. In the delicate skin around the eyes the allergic substances in nail varnish can excite redness, swelling and itching. Many women coming into an allergy clinic complaining of swellings round the eyes are surprised to be told they are allergic to their nail varnish.

Cosmetics can also cause allergies due to the perfume they contain. In some people perfume irritates the skin so that it produces more pigment than normal and brown patches appear. It is most common down the side of the face, near the forehead and over the cheekbone, but it may extend on to the neck. It can take up to a year to disappear and you must avoid the sun if you do not want the patches to go darker.

You will not go far wrong if you stick to cosmetics that are pure, simple and inexpensive. This does not mean joining the fashion for products which claim to be made entirely from natural extracts. Objective evidence is yet to be seen for the magic properties of zest of lemon, juice of cucumber or oil of avocado. If baby lotion is good enough for baby skin, it follows that it should be good enough for adult skin.

Just as important as what you put on your skin is the way you put it on. Every

The directions your fingers should follow when applying or removing make-up

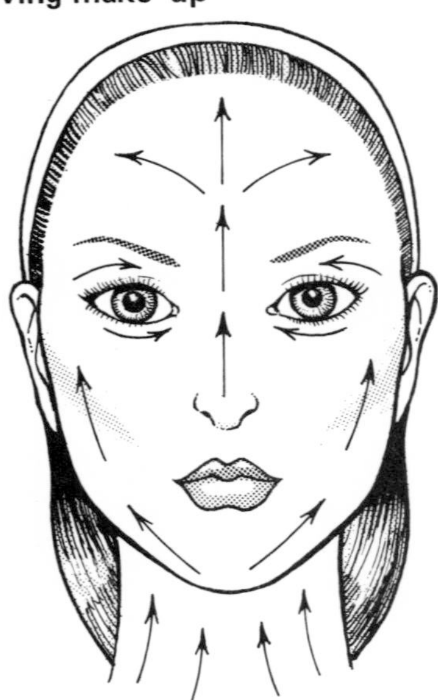

The main point about beauty routines is that the fingers should move over the skin in an upward direction. Take great care when massaging particularly delicate skin, e.g. that around the eyes.

day of your life from the age of say, sixteen, you put on and take off make-up maybe three times a day. Cumulatively, that is an awful lot of massage and you can do your skin a lot of good by massaging it properly and a lot of harm by doing it badly. You should always massage your face in a way that minimizes and counteracts the ageing effects of gravity's pull, by following the movements which are shown in the diagram opposite.

Hair and nails

The skin has two important appendages – the hair and the nails. Both have living and growing roots but at the point where we can see and treat the hair and nails their cells are dead. Long hair has been dead for three years or more. This fact goes a long way to explaining why potions applied to the hair cannot radically change its constitution, except transiently. The time when you can influence the health of your hair is while it is growing. It grows from the hair follicle at a rate of about 0.2 to 0.4 millimetres per week and its quality is a reflection of your state of general health and nutrition at that time. A diet for healthy hair and nails should be balanced and contain foods with plenty of vitamin A, such as liver, fish and milk.

We have several different types of hair: scalp hair, eyebrow and eyelash hair, beard hair, 'secondary sexual' hair – for example in the armpits, in the genital area and on the chest of men – and very small hairs that cover most parts of the skin except the palms of the hands and the soles of the feet. These hairs grow

A hair follicle magnified

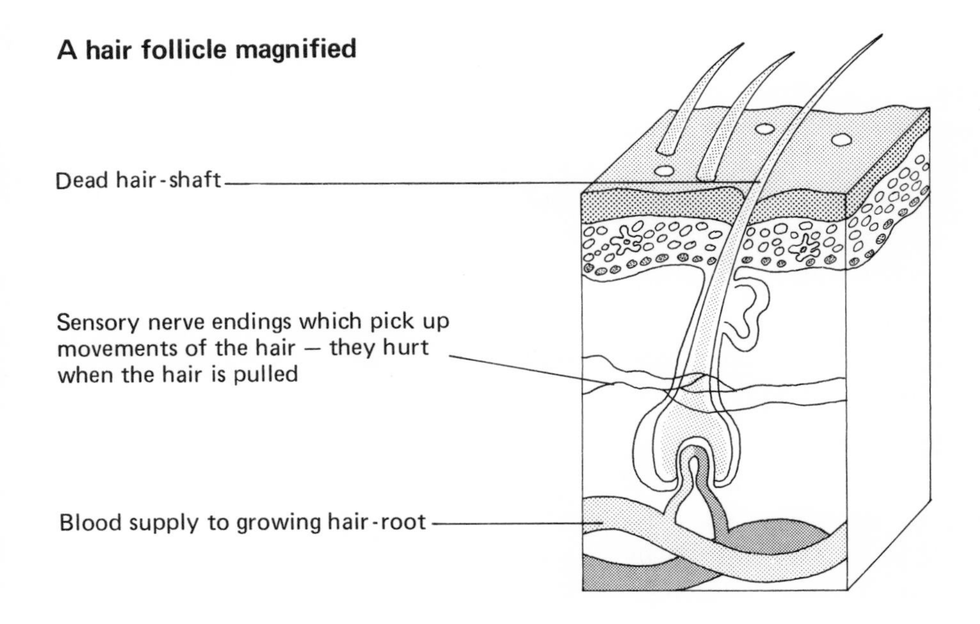

away from the midline. Given a solitary finger you can tell if it is from the right or left hand by examining the direction of the hair growth; looking at the finger with the fingernail pointing towards you, it is a right finger if the hair is growing towards your left, and vice versa.

The growth of these types of hair is controlled in different ways. It is interesting that male hormones are responsible for both hair growth in the beard area and lack of growth (baldness) on the scalp. Hair growth, particularly of the scalp, goes through cycles of activity and rest, but synchronously, so that some hairs are growing while others are resting. This means that hair loss is hardly noticeable, except if an event pushes all the hair into one phase as pregnancy does. Many women notice that at any time between three and eighteen months after their baby is born they suffer frightening hair loss. This is normal and the thickness of the hair will return in due course, though it may take as long as two or three years.

There are a few myths about hair which should be dispelled:

DANDRUFF: Dandruff is the natural scaling of the scalp as it sheds its dead uppermost layers. The hair strands tend to trap the scales and they may pile up. It is not therefore either a disease or an infection but merely a variation of normal. It follows that you need not use a medicated shampoo to get rid of it. Anything which irritates the scalp like vigorous brushing and massaging will only encourage more dandruff as producing scales faster is the only way that the scalp can protect itself. (For treatment see **Dandruff**, p. 159.)

SHAMPOOS: Some of the anti-dandruff shampoos contain an ingredient which is irritating if used too frequently so this kind of shampoo should be restricted to once a fortnight. The basic rule with shampoos is to use the mildest one you can find – a baby shampoo is very suitable. In a dermatology clinic in which I worked we used a carpet shampoo: whereas most people are prepared to take risks with their hair, they are not prepared to take the same risk with their best worsted Wilton carpet, nor were the manufacturers, so it was an extremely mild shampoo. We used to recommend a teaspoonful of the shampoo in a glassful of water used once on the hair.

CONDITIONERS: Conditioners of any kind, no matter how effective they may appear to be immediately after washing, can only have a temporary softening effect on dead hair.

WASHING THE HAIR: Most hair, even if it is fine and dry, benefits from being washed fairly frequently. Most dermatologists advocate washing the hair every three or four days or so. The hair and scalp should not be vigorously rubbed. Rubbing the scalp only irritates it and stimulates the production of grease and dandruff. The shampoo should be gently massaged into the hair, left in contact with it for no more than two minutes, then rinsed off. Hair, if anything, should be underwashed, never overwashed. Usually one wash is enough regardless of manufacturers' instructions. Any serious scalp or skin problem should of course be treated by your doctor.

The nails grow from the live nail-plate at the rate of 1 to 2 millimetres per month and are dead by the time they emerge from the cuticle. They are even more sensitive barometers of physical and emotional health than hair. A crisis of any sort, be it a serious illness or period of stress, can show up in the nails as a transverse ridge in their horny surface. Several illnesses leave tell-tale signs in the nails and a favourite examination topic for medical students is the diseases that may be diagnosed by examination of the nails – psoriasis, iron-deficiency anaemia and liver disease being but three. (See also **Nails**, pp. 184–5.)

Cellulite

Cellulite is a subject often written and talked about. Having studied very carefully a monumental Swiss document about cellulite, I am none the wiser. Cellulite is not a medical term, it describes no medical condition known to doctors, and I have yet to see a description of it that explains it in medically accepted terms.

Cellulite is the word that has been coined to describe dimpling of fat. It is seen most often on the thighs, but it can appear wherever there is too much fat under the skin, like the upper arm. It is confined to females and occurs rarely in young ones and rarely in thin ones. It is a condition, generally speaking, of obese middle-aged women, and is variously described as being due to abnormalities of fat metabolism or abnormal collections of fluid. The use of the word abnormal suggests that normality might be reinstated by some form of treatment, and such is female vanity that treatment is demanded. An irresistible demand will always find suppliers, hence the numerous offers of numerous treatments.

Dimpling of the skin over excessive layers of fat is not, however, abnormal, it is a variant of normal. No amount of massage, electrical stimulation or medication will correct it. It can often disappear though, if the cellulite lady loses sufficient weight to slim down her thighs and upper arms. But this too often requires more perseverance than most cellulite sufferers possess.

pH-controlled beauty aids

One new idea that has been introduced into the beauty business in the last few years and is scientifically very attractive, is the idea of pH control. The 'pH' is a measure of the acidity or alkalinity of things. The natural pH of the skin is well on the acid side. The acidity results from the secretion of sebum which contains several natural acids, and it is necessary for the skin's health, growth, smooth surface and for the suppression of bacterial multiplication. This applies to hair too. Nearly all the substances used to wash the skin and hair contain detergents which are strongly alkaline and this profoundly disturbs the health, ecology, appearance and feel of the skin. Any cleanser which has a similar pH to the skin and hair (often described as 'pH buffered') is therefore preferable to a strongly alkaline one.

Electrolysis

Electrolysis can be used in the treatment of facial and unwanted body hair. The aim of electrolysis is to kill the growing hair root. During treatment a fine needle carrying an electric current results in the shrivelling of the hair root. Usually only a few hairs are treated at a time – according to your stoicism. In good hands the treatment should be virtually painless. Only seek treatment from an accredited practitioner – in the wrong hands scarring can occur. Electrolysis is available on the National Health for some patients through your local GP and consultant dermatologist.

Massage and electrical stimulation

If you have a massage to make you feel good then you probably will not be disappointed, but if you have a massage to lose weight I can guarantee that you will. Your masseur may lose weight, not you. Fat cannot be rubbed away by hands, machines, moving belts or bumping rollers. Nor can it be removed, as though by magic, with electrical stimulating pads that make the muscles contract. A muscle has to contract many times against a force for a considerable period of time to use up sufficient energy to show as weight loss. Exercise, while essential for keeping you fit, is a very inefficient way of burning off excess calories: it takes over an hour digging in the garden or two hours walking to burn up the calories in a four-ounce bar of chocolate. The best answer is not to take them in.

I am opposed to all forms of apparatus or techniques which claim to make you lose weight while you do nothing yourself. The quickest way to show a drop in your weight is to lose water. You can achieve this with drugs (diuretics) or by wearing a garment which makes you sweat or by lowering your intake. As soon as you go back to normal your body will restore its natural water balance over the next few days and you will put on those pounds you took off without being able to do anything about it.

The beauty game is encouraged because people are made to feel inadequate for not looking the way the ad-men would have them believe they ought to look, so the search is on for easy ways out, for short cuts, for overnight solutions and miracle changes. Well, they do not exist. The maintenance of a slim figure needs constant vigilance, keeping a good skin in good condition means regular care. Like all other aspects of staying fit and healthy, it requires effort, not from others or machines or bottles or jars, but from *you*. You have to work at it. If you cannot be bothered, keep your expectations low and confine them to your own, not the advertisers'.

10 Can Modern Medicine Learn from Ancient Remedies?

Herbal remedies used in the past

Sickness and disease have always affected human beings. In parallel, human beings have always desired to replace sickness with health; they have always had the desire to heal. This desire to heal is a characteristic which makes us different from all other animals.

Medical traditions first began in China where it was the custom to pay a doctor to keep a patient well and to stop paying him when the patient became ill. Chinese medicine along with most other forms of ancient medicine relied on the healing properties of herbs and plants. In the very beginning herbal medicine was a hit-and-miss affair, and only after generations of observations was a particular herb associated with a particular effect in a particular disease. Remedies were handed down through families and were not the prerogative of a designated 'healer'. Practically every household had its own pharmacopoeia of favourite teas and tonics obtained from the roots and bark and leaves of plants. This form of medicine was necessarily empirical with no attempt at diagnosis – quite the opposite methodology of medicine as it is practised today!

In the light of present knowledge, many of the ancient remedies may have had no scientific basis at all. For instance, there are hundreds of medicinal plants that are supposed to be good for diabetes but not one of them is used by a reputable physician. There is no doubt that many folk remedies have a demonstrable biological action, but the results are very often so unpredictable that today's doctors are unwilling to work within so great a margin of error.

Folk medicine is not without its triumphs. Cleopatra was known to use the juice of a succulent called *Aloe vera* which has recently been shown by the University of Pennsylvania to be more effective in treating radiation burns than any other available preparation.

The Egyptians were also on to the medicinal properties of cabbage. They ate the seed to prevent intoxication. It would appear that the Romans, too, had latched on to cabbage as a pick-me-up. Here is a quotation from Cato: 'If you wish to drink much at a banquet, before dinner dip cabbage in vinegar and eat as much as you will. When you have dined, eat five leaves. The cabbage will make you as fit as if you had had nothing and you can drink as much as you will.' To this day sauerkraut juice is still a popular remedy for hangovers. It was left to the eminent American chemist, Dr William Shive, to provide a scientific basis for the apparent potency of cabbage in warding off the effects of alcohol. He extracted an amino acid from cabbage juice and he used it for the treatment of alcoholism with good results.

As with cabbage, it may be centuries before a plant yields all its mysteries. There are several other examples of well-known plant remedies which were not fully understood until they were analyzed by methods which only became available as modern technology advanced. For example, in the early 1950s scientists investigated for the first time the ancient Hindu snake root which had been used for centuries in the treatment of insanity. The active ingredient was extracted from the root and turned out to be the first modern tranquillizer, reserpine. It was also found to be effective in the treatment of high blood-pressure and for many years doctors used this drug as the treatment of choice.

The Mexican yam gave up its secrets in the 1940s. It had been noted that native women chewed on the root of the yam daily as they believed that the root prevented them from becoming pregnant, and so it did. It was discovered that a complex steroid substance called diosgenin could be extracted from the root of the yam. This steroid is the starting substance from which something like 10 million chemicals can be made. The isolation of diosgenin from the Mexican yam led to the synthesis of other steroid substances which have completely revolutionized medicine: cortisone, for example, which is the chief substance of the most potent group of anti-inflammatory medicines yet known for the treatment of such disorders as arthritis and asthma; possibly more important, because of the impact that they had on society, were the synthetic female sex hormones which heralded the advent of the oral contraceptive pill; yet other potent steroid substances which could be chemically adapted to make them active when applied to the skin for the treatment of serious skin disorders.

But it was when a particular disease became a world-wide hazard that the age-old remedy for it became a matter of international importance. The disease was malaria and the treatment was cinchona bark. The first reference to the medicinal properties of the cinchona tree occurs in a chronicle written in South America about the middle of the seventeenth century: 'A tree grows which they call the fever tree in the country of Loxa, whose bark is the colour of cinnamon. When made into a powder amounting to the weight of two small silver coins and given as a beverage, it cures the fevers and tertians. It has produced miraculous cures in Lima.'

At about the same time in Rome, experiments with the 'bark of barks' were found to be very successful. It was not only non-toxic but it was also the most effective treatment ever tried for the fevers then so common in Rome. After its successful use on an ecclesiastical gentleman high in the Vatican, the Peruvian bark came to be known as the 'powder of the most eminent cardinal'.

In England the bark was introduced in 1654 when the ague covered the country. Oliver Cromwell contracted the fever but of course it was out of the question for him to use the 'powder of the most eminent cardinal', and so he succumbed to malaria in 1658. Throughout history, malaria has dogged the steps of military men. Alexander the Great died of it in 323 BC. George Washington caught malaria during the American War of Independence, but his life, unlike those of thousands of his soldiers, was saved by the use of cinchona powder. During the Second World War, cinchona bark products were still the only treatment for malaria available to the army, and supplies of medicines became critical as army operations entered areas where malaria was endemic. The situation became so bad that there was a period during the war when the American chiefs of staff believed that the US army would be defeated unless huge quantities of quinine (the active ingredient in cinchona bark) could be made available to the army. In 1944 two American scientists found a laboratory method to duplicate the chemical structure of quinine and so made possible the first production of synthetic anti-malarials.

Chaulmoogra seeds were recommended for the treatment of leprosy in the oldest Chinese and Indian medical writings. There is an Indian legend about King Rama of Benares who developed leprosy and hid himself in the jungle where he lived on a diet of berries and herbs. His diet fortuitously included the seeds of the chaulmoogra tree; he found his symptoms subsiding until eventually he was cured. One day as he was walking through the forest, the legend goes on, he heard the screaming of a frightened girl from a nearby cave. King Rama went into the cave and rescued the girl, Pya, from a tiger who was threatening her. Pya had once been a beautiful princess but she was now disfigured by leprosy. King Rama collected the seeds of the chaulmoogra tree and gave them to Pya as medicine. Her leprosy too disappeared and they were married, raised sixteen sets of twins, and lived happily ever after.

There is a recipe which was in existence more than three thousand years ago which states that chaulmoogra oil is very efficacious in leprosy. It is given in doses of ten to twenty drops after meals and it may also be used externally on the affected parts. It was advocated that the treatment should be continued for at least three months. Over the centuries medical science could not improve very much on this. The regimen employed at the US National Centre for the Treatment of Leprosy in the late 1940s was as follows: treatment usually began with gelatin capsules, containing five drops of chaulmoogra oil, taken daily after meals; the dosage was increased until the patient's tolerance was reached. Chaulmoogra was also frequently used locally in ointments or liniments.

The English country garden, too, has played its part in the history of plant medicine by making what is probably the single most important contribution to the treatment of heart disease. It started in a Shropshire hedgerow with the foxglove. William Withering was a young doctor when he wrote the following:

> In the year 1775 my opinion was asked concerning a family receipt for the cure of dropsy.* I was told that it had long been kept a secret by an old woman in Shropshire, who had sometimes made cures after the more regular practitioners had failed. I was informed also that the effects produced were violent vomiting and purging; the diuretic effect seemed to have been overlooked. This medication was composed of twenty or more different herbs; but it was not very difficult for one conversant in these subjects to perceive that the active herb could be no other than Foxglove.

We are all beholden to William Withering for not dismissing the family remedy. He continued to gain experience with the use of foxglove preparations and he became familiar with the dosage and the side effects that it caused. He was one of the few doctors who did, and much of his work was scorned by his fellows. With only minor refinements digitalis, obtained from the leaves and flowers of foxgloves, is still the standard drug used in the treatment of many forms of heart disease to this day.

Not all folk remedies have stood the test of time so well. It is difficult to rationalize the use of beetroot juice for the treatment of baldness, or vinegar and brown paper for the alleviation of bronchitis. It also stretches the credulity to understand how the two favourite ingredients of herbal pharmacopoeia, nettle juice and garlic, can exert healing effects in so many diverse conditions. In the case of nettle juice, anaemia, acne, arthritis, baldness, chilblains, diarrhoea, dropsy, obesity, and shingles. In the case of garlic, arthritis, blood poisoning, cholera, diphtheria, influenza, goitre, insomnia, laryngitis, neuralgia and piles.

And with the best will in the world it is difficult to see the medical rationale of the following treatments: placing the feet in hot water with a couple of spoonfuls of mustard powder for a stroke; giving asparagus to bed-wetters; drinking rose-petal tea for brain fatigue; applying a little fresh cream to a cut or wound; taking warm baths and a brisk walk before breakfast for depression; taking daily baths for lung complaints; washing with cold marigold tea as a restorative for the sexual organs; placing a leaf of fresh cabbage on the side to relieve a stitch; taking a large dessertspoonful of pure honey and a pinch of cinnamon in warm, but not boiled, milk as a tranquillizer (Valium users please note!!).

The truth and falsehood of some old wives' cures

Well, which of grannie's preventatives, restoratives and cures have a glimmer of truth in them?

* Dropsy is swollen ankles due to the pooling of fluid in the dependent parts of the body and occurs when the pumping action of a failing heart is insufficient to keep the fluid circulating.

Vinegar on a wasp sting: Good idea. A wasp sting is alkaline. The acid in the vinegar neutralizes this and reduces irritation. NB Soda is used for a bee sting.

Soda on an ant bite: Good idea. Ants inject formic acid into the skin and soda neutralizes the acid thereby reducing irritation.

Carrots help you to see in the dark: Half true. Carrots contain a lot of vitamin A which is necessary for the health of the cells in the retina which enable us to see in the dark. But eating more carrots will not improve their health. It is said that this was a rumour put around in the war to make the Germans think that our fighter pilots had exceptional night vision.

Bread crusts make your hair curly: Not true. A ruse to get you to eat bread crusts.

An apple a day keeps the doctor away: Not true. Apples are no better for you than any other fruit. In fact they are less good for you than fruits containing lots of vitamin C like oranges or vegetables like tomatoes. They are better than a fattening dessert though.

Feed a cold and starve a fever: Not true. When you have a fever your metabolism is speeded up and you need more calories not less, otherwise you start to burn up your own precious proteins to provide calories. If you have a fever you must never neglect to drink plenty of fluids which are lost by the pint if you are sweating.

Gelatin makes your nails grow: Wrong. Your nails are part of your heredity, just like the colour of your eyes. No food can make for one particular part of the body. It is circulated and spread throughout the whole of the body and does not concentrate in one area. So it is pointless to take something by mouth, such as gelatin, in the hope that it will make for your nails alone.

Cooking in cast-iron pots will give you iron: True. Research has shown that eggs scrambled for three minutes in an iron pan have more than twice as much iron as those scrambled for three minutes in any other sort of pan. And if you cook a stew in an iron pot, say for three hours, it will have as much as thirty times more iron in it than if it is cooked in a pan made of another metal. Some nutritionists say that women especially should supplement their diet by cooking whenever possible in cast-iron pans. However, don't forget the foods which are rich in iron, such as meat, liver and green vegetables.

You can charm away warts: True. Any wart charm has a good chance of working if the wart has been present for eighteen months or longer. The reason is this: the warts are caused by a virus and it takes the body about eighteen months to build up its own antibodies to that virus and kill it off. When the virus is dead the wart will disappear. Now the body will do this of its own accord. Since nine out of ten warts disappear eighteen months to two years after they first appear your witchcraft should be accredited to the body's own defence mechanism.

Masturbation can make you blind: Totally untrue.

Drink a bottle of gin for an abortion: Partly true. More true when gin was less well-refined than it now is. If you and the baby are healthy, nothing will shift the baby other than mechanical intervention. If, on the other hand, you are in a low state of health and the baby is not normal and is insecurely implanted in the uterus, the gin (more particularly the impurities in the gin) may stimulate sufficiently strong contractions to expel the baby.

An apple or a raw carrot last thing at night will clean your teeth: Wrong. Apples and carrots are no more cariogenic than other foods but they are no less so, and have no cleaning effect.

Put a piece of mouldy bacon on a cut: Good. Mould on the bacon is a relative of the mould that produces penicillin and although our grannies did not know it they were using 'antibiotics' for the first time.

Put a burn in cold water: Good. Burnt skin usually dies. You can stop it from dying by slowing down its metabolism and we all know that metabolism is slower when the temperature drops. So if you keep your burn cold you will reduce the likelihood of getting a blister or having severe damage to your skin and you will also reduce the pain.

Steak on a black eye: Questionable. The theory behind this remedy is that there are enzymes in muscle (lean steak) which in certain circumstances can reduce inflammation and swelling and so prevent bruising. The scientific drawback to this theory is that the chemical molecules of most of the enzymes are too complex to penetrate the skin. You'll benefit more from eating the steak.

Butterballs rolled in sugar for a sore throat: Possibly good. The butter slides down easily and keeps the sugar in its crystalline form. The crystals tend to abrade the sore throat and remove infected debris and pus.

Dock leaves on nettle stings: Good remedy. Dock leaves contain a natural antihistamine substance which to some extent neutralizes the histamine released into the skin (which causes the itching) when the sting enters the skin. The leaves should be crushed so that the sap is released. Bicarbonate of soda is also good.

Key or ice down the back for nosebleeds: Bad remedy for nose bleeds (see pp. 185–6). Good remedy for hiccups which may stop abruptly with a shock.

Head between knees for fainting: Good remedy. Keeps blood supply to brain going (see pp. 166–7).

Oil of cloves for toothache: Good temporarily, because of anaesthetic properties. Bad if used too frequently because damages the gums (see p. 199).

Witchhazel for bruises: Good. Helps to reduce the swelling.

Copper bracelets for rheumatism: Very questionable. Started because Dutch settlers in Rhodesia noticed natives who wore copper ornaments never got rheumatism. Despite many keen advocates, never proven. Believers say effect linked to vibrations emitted by copper. It sounds farfetched but who knows?

Rubbing a stye with an eighteen-carat gold ring: Not true.

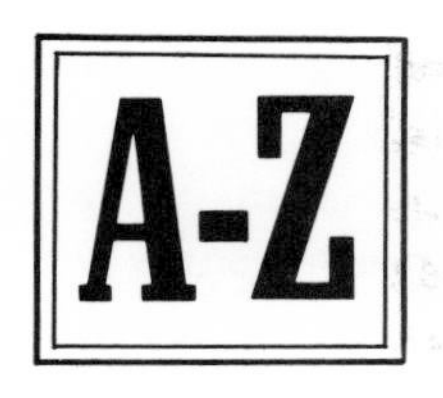

# of Common Medical Complaints and How to Treat Them

This section is not meant to be exhaustive. I have tried to restrict the list of problems to those which are common and have purposely excluded rare complaints. The section does not include conditions where there is little first aid or self help that you can administer, where the treatment is for a skilled medical practitioner only. The aim is to free you from old wives' remedies, give you a background which will encourage you to use your own common sense in treating everyday medical problems but never to overreach yourself, and to consult your doctor if you are in any doubt whatsoever.

The section is also intended to give you guidelines as to what you can do in certain emergencies while you are waiting for expert help to arrive. These are not presented *en bloc* but are listed alphabetically so the emergency treatment for burns comes under *B*, suspected fracture under *F* and wounds which are bleeding profusely under *B*. Certain emergency first-aid procedures are included even though they are primarily the job of a doctor. They are included because if you try to perform them, even imperfectly, you may save a life, whereas if you do not a life may be lost while you are waiting for help. Such manoeuvres include the kiss of life, external cardiac massage and tracheotomy.

Nearly all the conditions discussed are ones affecting adults and older children. I have dealt with illnesses relating particularly to babies and young children in my previous book, *Miriam Stoppard's Book of Babycare* (Weidenfeld and Nicolson, 1977). There is no discussion at all of psychiatric complaints as I feel that brief written advice on this subject is always inadequate.

Viruses and bacteria

In the following pages I frequently refer to bacteria and viruses as a cause of illness. It is important to understand the difference between the two when considering the treatment of ailments. We usually think of bacteria and viruses in the context of infection, but not all are pathogenic (cause illness). Our skin is swarming with bacteria, the flora (bacterial population) of the mouth contains half a dozen species, and in the gut many different varieties live in perfect harmony. Bacteria cause disease if they produce powerful poisons (toxins) and increase rapidly in number. Most of the bacteria that harmlessly inhabit parts of the body do not make powerful toxins and numerically are kept in check by the presence of other bacteria which are competing for nourishment.

Bacteria are very simple single-celled plants and as such can multiply quickly. Pathogenic bacteria are passed on by touch or by contaminated foodstuffs. They are killed by bacteriocidal antibiotics, e.g. penicillin, and are prevented from multiplying by bacteriostatic antibiotics, e.g. sulphonamides. If they are exposed to a low concentration of an antibiotic they are stimulated to throw up new strains (mutants) which are resistant to that antibiotic.

A virus is the smallest living thing known. It is virtually a chain of DNA (deoxyribonucleic acid) which is the key chemical in any living cell. Viruses cannot live unsupported. They will only survive if they are inside a living cell. They reproduce themselves very quickly and may also change their own structure. Hence we may have one variety of Asian flu at the beginning of winter and six more 'relatives' by the spring. This accounts for the lack of protection from flu vaccines – you may be infected by a different strain of virus from that against which you were vaccinated.

Drug-taking

We are the generation of drug-takers. Never before have so many diverse remedies been sought from bottles, both prescribed and self-administered. Their availability no doubt contributes to the easy-going attitude to such medicines as pain-killers, tranquillizers and sleeping pills. Many, of course, are needed but only rarely in the long term. If the need is chronic then expert guidance should be given. In many instances drugs are being abused or carelessly used. In the main pain-killers, tranquillizers and sleeping pills should be used to get over a bad patch and to help form new habits; otherwise they frequently become habit-forming themselves. You should especially try to avoid long-term medication and only take medicines when you really need them. If you find yourself having recourse to any medicine, even an antacid, for longer than a week, you should consult your doctor.

It is particularly important to avoid taking drugs in the first three months of pregnancy: never take anything, not even aspirin which we tend to forget is a powerful drug, without consulting your doctor. And never give a child patent medicines for more than a day except under supervision by your doctor.

The careless use of antibiotics is also to be deprecated. The more often antibiotics are used without just cause or improperly, the greater the likelihood of resistant strains of bacteria developing. We then find ourselves in the dangerous situation of not having antibiotics which can kill resistant strains. A few basic rules:

1 Do not expect your doctor to give you antibiotics for every minor infection.

2 Take antibiotics *exactly* as instructed, particularly with regard to frequency and time interval.

3 Always, always, always finish the course.

4 Dispose of old tablets, capsules and syrups so they cannot be found by children.

5 Never self-medicate with antibiotics.

Analgesics

We can resort so readily to analgesics (pain-killers) that there is a tendency to discount them as active drugs. Most of them are powerful and effective but can have side effects which range from merely irritating to life-threatening.

ASPIRIN Used correctly it is one of the most useful remedies in the pharmacopaeia. It and its derivatives can be used in many surprising though simple ways: as an ointment to get rid of hard skin; as a gargle with antiseptic properties; as a liniment for sore muscles; as an inhalant for inflamed bronchial tubes; as an analgesic tablet (preferably the soluble form). Aspirin is used by doctors in high doses for its anti-inflammatory properties and is particularly useful in rheumatoid arthritis and rheumatic fever affecting the heart. The analgesic effect of one dose lasts four to six hours.

The commonest side effect is gastric irritation which manifests itself as dyspepsia or, rarely, bleeding. In very high doses you get deafness and ringing in the ears and an overdose may be fatal in a few hours because the aspirin deranges the mechanism which controls the acidity and alkalinity of the body. You should not take any medicines containing aspirin for a hangover because of possible gastric irritation.

PARACETAMOL (Acctominophen in USA) It is a marginally weaker analgesic drug than aspirin but in most instances it is worth sacrificing the efficacy for greater safety. It does have some fairly rare side effects but it is largely free of gastric irritation which means that people with peptic ulcers can take it. It is also safer than aspirin for infants and is available as a syrup. The effect of one dose lasts four to six hours.

CODEINE It is a very powerful centrally acting (it acts on the pain centre) analgesic. It will also act on the cough centre in the brain and is a fairly common constituent of cough medicines. Although its effect lasts only four or five hours, it is capable of relieving all but the most severe pain. Side effects with codeine are not a rarity: the commonest is constipation because it damps down the movements of the bowel (indeed it can be used as a treatment for diarrhoea), and headache and dizziness are not infrequent. Codeine should not be taken on a regular basis unless under the supervision of a doctor. Even though it is only a distant relative of morphine it has to be handled with care.

PHENACETIN It used to be a common ingredient in pain-killing preparations, but because it has a harmful effect on the kidneys there are now strict rules about its use. If you are buying a patent pain-killer, have a look at the ingredients and if the preparation contains phenacetin, it is better to avoid it unless your doctor approves of its use. Nearly all the cases of kidney damage reported with phenacetin are in patients who took the substance over a long period of time. You will probably not come to any harm if you use it in the short term.

How to handle your doctor

Being a doctor myself, and being aware of the niceties of what is considered an ethical code of conduct between doctors, I cannot help being aware of certain expectations which a doctor has of his patients' conduct and vice versa. I make no judgement of them but hazard a few suggestions which, in my experience, help to keep your relationship with your doctor a happy one.

1 If you want her to visit you, telephone the surgery before 9 a.m. so that your doctor can plan her day.

2 If you suspect you may have to call your doctor in the night, warn the surgery so that your doctor can decide whether to visit you earlier.

3 With a sick child under two years old, alert your doctor if you are worried; do not wait until you present her with an emergency.

4 Do not consult another doctor without telling your own doctor first; this is not just professional courtesy, it is in your own interests because your GP may have medical information that a second doctor would wish to have while assessing your case.

5 Some women find it difficult to discuss female complaints with a man and vice versa. In this instance the initiative lies with the woman. Male doctors are never embarrassed by such conversations but will appreciate a woman's reticence. You will be avoiding your responsibility if you are not honest with your doctor so do not lose your nerve and mislead him with a minor or fictitious complaint.

6 Do not be over fussy about yourself or your family, or hypochondriacal. It is not the best way to gain co-operation from anyone and you may cry wolf once too often.

7 Ask your doctor for information about yourself, your illness and your treatment. Your questions will almost certainly be welcomed. As a bright-eyed junior doctor, most willing to fulfil a patient's right to have things explained to them, I quickly became disillusioned with the small number who reciprocated my interest.

8 Do not always expect a prescription from your doctor. Not all complaints need medicine and quite often medical advice is sufficient.

9 Do not expect your doctor to be infallible. Like every other person your doctor is human and your expectations should be realistic, not only in terms of her fallibility but also her preoccupations and moods.

As a patient you have certain rights: to a second opinion; to consult a specialist privately; and to leave your doctor's panel.

It is understandable that a doctor may view the request for a second opinion as a criticism of her own ability and you should be sympathetic to this professional pride by approaching the subject frankly and diplomatically. If you express your concerns honestly, most doctors will be more than happy to reassure you by arranging an appointment with another doctor, perhaps a partner. If your doctor will not do this, I would guess that your relationship is not a good one and you would both probably welcome a change.

If you introduce your wish to see a private specialist in the way I have just described, you will probably find your doctor most co-operative. If you go to see a specialist without telling your doctor, and especially if you feel you would rather not discuss the matter, then it suggests that you and your doctor do not get on too well.

You should never change your doctor without prior discussion, and agreement if possible. Like any other person who performs a service for you, your doctor should have the opportunity to put things right if you are dissatisfied and to agree to a parting of the ways if your differences are irreconcilable.

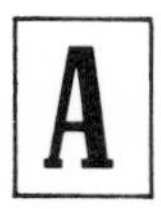

Abscess An abscess is a collection of pus. Pus is composed of dead tissue, dead white blood cells and the dead bacteria which were the source of the infection. An abscess usually exhibits the four classical signs of inflammation: redness, pain, swelling and heat. A small localized abscess, for example, a boil in the skin, will cause nothing more than local symptoms. But a large internal abscess, say of the liver or kidney, will cause a very high, swinging temperature and extreme illness.

The universal treatment for an abscess, once the pus is formed, is to open it and allow the pus to drain. You can encourage pus to form, or 'come to a head', with hot poultices; for instance, of Fuller's earth which retains heat. With a small superficial abscess in the skin or gum ('gum boil'), a sharp instrument such as a needle, sterilized for a minute or so in a flame, can be used to drain the pus. The abscess is punctured and the hole made large enough to allow the pus to drain out freely. Pus may be pressed out very gently. An abscess should never be squeezed forcibly as this may spread the infection into surrounding healthy tissues. Dress the abscess each day by bathing with a weak antiseptic solution and covering with a dry dressing. Remove a dry dressing by bathing it until it comes unstuck. A large or internal abscess will probably need antibiotic treatment by mouth as well as surgical drainage. An abscess which fails to respond to your own treatment within twenty-four hours needs expert attention.

Acne Skin complaints, especially of the face, are most common during adolescence when blackheads, pimples and acne make their appearance. One of the causes is the outpouring of sexual hormones which occurs as a person enters the early teens and, though it is caused by an excessive quantity of the male hormone, androgen, it is common to both sexes. An excess of androgens is produced by girls as well as boys during their adolescent years.

The basic skin lesion in acne is the blackhead, which is caused by the blockage of a sebaceous gland. The sebaceous gland becomes blocked because the high levels of androgens cause the cells at the neck of the gland to increase in number and close off the opening, preventing the escape of sebum on to the surface of the skin. The sebum collects behind the blockage, the gland swells and eventually bursts. Sebum, when liberated into the lower layers of the skin, is an extreme irritant and inflammation is set up which becomes secondarily infected. The whole area swells – the acne nodule – and becomes infected – the acne pustule.

Most acne clears as the patient gets older. It is not known why one individual should suffer from acne and another should not, but it is probably due to the sensitivity of the sebaceous glands to high levels of androgens. Many women experience acne in the week prior to menstruation and again this is due to high circulating levels of progesterone which in a metabolic sense is a close cousin of androgen.

Blackheads may be gently squeezed after bathing the skin with warm water, thereby opening up the pores and allowing the plug of cells to escape more easily. Acne pustules may also be gently burst and the pus wiped away with a small piece of cotton wool soaked in a mild antiseptic solution. With these exceptions, a golden rule for everyone is *don't squeeze spots.*

There are very few cases of adult acne but they tend to be severe and require rigorous specialized treatment usually only available in hospital departments – treatments such as ultra-violet radiation or surgical abrasion.

Everyone can do certain things to help minimize acne:

1 Wash the skin at least twice a day with an antiseptic soap. This should be done by making a lather in the palm of the hand and gently massaging the lather into the skin for a minute or two and then rinsing off. The skin should never be rubbed hard and never abrade.

2 The application of an antiseptic lotion, such as pHisoHex, to reduce the numbers of bacteria on the skin which can cause secondary infection of the acne nodules.

3 The use of antiseptic cream – the best ones are only available on prescription – which are used at least night and morning and, in girls, under make-up.

4 Expose oneself as much as possible to sunlight (though not necessarily ultra-violet lamps). Mild sunburn causes peeling of the skin and this unblocks the sebaceous glands and helps to prevent and cure acne.

5 Diet has been shown to have nothing to do with acne so there is no point in avoiding rich foods like chocolate and fatty foods on that account.

6 Severe acne should alway be treated by a physician.

7 When I used to do an acne clinic I always advised teenage girls to wear a fairly heavily tinted make-up, very often to the horror of their mothers. Contrary to old wives' tales, make-up cannot block the pores, in fact nothing can block the pores of the skin and a heavily tinted make-up will cover up the colour, and, to a certain extent, the disfigurement caused by acne nodules and acne pustules. This camouflage can greatly improve a girl's morale and if her morale is improved, she will feel better and look better and her acne actually will *be* better. This aspect of treating acne is extremely important as demoralization and depression can itself worsen the acne.

Adenoids Adenoids are glands situated at the very back of the nose and, along with the tonsils, they undergo enlargement if a child has infection of the ear, nose and throat. Because of their position, adenoids can block the nasal air passages and a child with chronically enlarged adenoids is often a mouth breather by day and a snorer by night.

Both the adenoids and the tonsils are part of the body's main defences against the entry of infection through the throat and nasal region; they trap and kill bacteria that invade these parts. The tonsils and adenoids are often called the 'watchdogs of the throat'. There is no need to remove either tonsils or adenoids unless they are a focus of recurrent infection leading to long-term suppuration of the ear or bronchial tubes or the formation of tonsillar abscesses. If this should occur then they should be removed in hospital by an ear, nose and throat specialist. If the adenoids are enlarged alone and are not associated with infection there is very little need for their removal. (See also **Tonsillitis**.)

Allergy Allergy is a state of altered sensitivity of the body which may affect different parts, e.g. the skin – hives; the eyes and nose – hay fever; the heart – rheumatic fever; the kidneys – nephritis, etc. There is a rule about allergy which states that *anyone* can become allergic to *anything* at *any time*. This means that you can drink milk for years and become allergic to it after thirty; you can become allergic to egg yolk after eating eggs for fifty years, and penicillin after taking it over sixty years. There is no hard and fast rule except that any substance can cause an allergy.

When I was learning dermatology I was told that there were only two substances to which one could not become allergic; these were gold and water. During my three years' apprenticeship I saw several cases of allergy to both these substances.

You only become allergic to something by being exposed to it *twice*. An allergy cannot develop on the *first* exposure to a foreign substance. An allergy will develop if the body recognizes a substance, usually protein, as foreign. Once recognized as foreign, the body produces antibodies which are capable of joining with, and neutralizing the foreign proteins (antigens) thereby rendering them harmless to the body. When this combination of antibody and antigen happens, however, irritating chemicals are liberated within the body which cause the different types of allergic reaction, for example: hives or urticaria, angioedema or swelling of the eyes and face and lips, anaphylaxis (a generalized allergic reaction throughout the body including the intestines, the heart and the blood-vessels which is extremely serious and may even cause death if not treated), asthma, eczema, some types of migraine, some types of ulcerative colitis.

The commonest allergies are fortunately not too serious and include allergies to food, frequently to fruit, such as strawberries, to fish, especially shell-fish, to meat, particularly tinned meats, and to nuts, coffee, tea and chocolate. It is a fairly simple matter to isolate the particular food which is causing an allergy by keeping a careful diary noting everything that you eat and then by skin testing in an allergy clinic with the suspected food. A positive skin test confirms that the food is the cause of the allergy. Treatment is a matter of avoiding it.

Treatment for an allergy of the skin does not involve putting anything on the skin itself, except something to cool it, like calamine lotion. The most effective treatment, antihistamines, must be taken internally usually three or five times a day. This will do a great deal to relieve the symptoms of the allergy. The treatment may need to be continued for several weeks. Unlike the earlier drugs the newest antihistamines are not soporific. Never put antihistamine creams on the skin – they can cause allergies!

More serious allergies require treatment with corticosteroids but this must be done under the supervision of a hospital specialist. If difficulty with breathing or loss of consciousness is part of an allergic attack, take the patient to hospital immediately.

Penicillin allergy is, unfortunately, quite common and the allergy extends to most relatives of penicillin. It therefore includes the newer penicillin-related antibiotics. Penicillin sensitivity can cause anaphylaxis – a type of allergic reaction where instead of one part of the body being affected as in hay fever or asthma or hives, many parts of the body react violently to the presence of the allergen. Anaphylaxis nearly always involves swelling of the eyes, mouth and face, swelling of the throat and inability to swallow, inflammation of the gastro-intestinal tract with abdominal pain and diarrhoea, a high temperature and rarely delirium, coma and even death. It can appear within seconds of exposure to the allergen and the person affected may collapse and lose consciousness. It constitutes a medical emergency and anyone suffering in this way should be taken immediately to hospital. Anaphylaxis is the most severe form of allergy and occurs in a very small minority of people who suffer from allergies. Apart from penicillin, the most commonly reported allergen which causes anaphylaxis is wasp stings. Anyone who is sensitive to penicillin or wasp stings should wear a disc stating this fact so that the proper steps can be taken rapidly should anaphylaxis occur.

Alopecia (Baldness) Though sufferers are reluctant to believe it, most cases of alopecia are simply variations of the norm. The most common form of alopecia is 'male baldness' which is deepening of the indentation of the hairline on both sides of the forehead. This is a secondary sexual charateristic of men, and a response of the scalp hair follicle to male sex hormones, so no treatment is indicated and no treatment will prevent it or cure it. No treatment should ever be given for it. In theory a hormone called an anti-androgen should treat baldness but none of these hormones have been fully tested. Baldness, which is a gradual extension of 'male baldness' and eventually involves the whole scalp, has the same cause and is also unresponsive to any local treatment.

Another form of alopecia which is physiological is that which occurs during pregnancy. Most women experience a thinning of the hair, especially just after the baby is born. The hair can fall for anything up to eighteen months and is very frightening indeed because the hair can become half as thick as it was before pregnancy. It will invariably recover but may be slow to do so, taking up to two or three years. The reason for this thinning of the hair during or just after pregnancy is that the pregnancy hormone, progesterone, drives all the hairs into a resting state simultaneously. They therefore fall at approximately the same time and this produces an exaggeration of what, under normal circumstances, is a very gradual, continuous process.

Alopecia areata is a form of baldness which appears as coin-shaped patches in the head where the hair follicle may die. If a hair follicle dies, and death can be diagnosed by a specialist using a magnifying glass, no treatment can bring it back to life. Alopecia areata is most commonly seen in middle-aged women of a nervous disposition and may appear after a shock or great emotional stress. It is difficult to treat and requires special treatment from a dermatologist. In no more than fifty per cent of the cases is the treatment successful.

The patent cures for baldness that one sees in newspapers have no relevance to or efficacy in the treatment of baldness.

Altitude sickness If you travel to a height of more than 3000 feet above sea level, you might well experience headaches, nausea, dizziness and a general feeling of being under the weather – the symptoms of altitude sickness. This is due to the effect of the change in altitude on the body and the exposure to a rarefied atmosphere where there is less oxygen than you are used to. The body can take up to three or four weeks to become accustomed to a lower concentration of oxygen in inhaled air. The immediate reaction to having less oxygen circulating in the blood are the symptoms already described. If the altitude is no more than, say, 6000 feet, the 'sickness' may go off in twenty-four to forty-eight hours, but at higher altitudes patients describe many other symptoms including depression, loss of appetite, inability to sleep, inability to concentrate, apathy and a general lassitude. After acclimatization, which may take several months, these symptoms nearly always subside and there is no treatment for this condition other than an explanation of why it occurs.

Amnesia We all suffer from amnesia to some degree and it usually gets worse as we get older – so-called senile amnesia which may affect many of us in a frighteningly premature way. The interesting thing about the amnesia of very old people is that they are forgetful only of recent events, so that while they cannot remember what they did this morning, they can remember with utmost clarity what they did fifty years ago.

After an accident accompanied by concussion, the patient may suffer what is called *retrograde amnesia*. Very often the longer the period of concussion, the longer the period of amnesia. Retrograde amnesia means that loss of memory extends backwards from the present into the past and may progress by extending further into the past. As the brain recovers from concussion, the memory gradually creeps back. Amnesia is rarely a permanent condition.

Anaemia The commonest form of anaemia is iron-deficiency anaemia, found mostly in women. This is not surprising because women lose at least .15 fluid ounces of blood with each menstrual period every month. Women who are menstruating need more iron in their diet than non-menstruating women, or men. The tendency of women to develop an iron-deficiency anaemia is greater during pregnancy when whatever the baby needs is taken from the mother. Because iron-deficiency anaemia is so common in pregnancy, iron supplements are routinely given to expectant mothers from the time pregnancy is diagnosed. With this prophylaxis iron-deficiency anaemia in pregnancy has become very rare.

A bleeding peptic ulcer may contribute to an iron-deficiency anaemia by the loss of only a few drops of blood every day. So you should seek diagnosis and active treatment of chronic dyspepsia and not rely on a packet of antacid tablets carried in your bag or pocket.

There are certain classical symptoms of iron-deficiency anaemia which can be spotted by observation alone: the conjunctivae of the eyes are pale (hence the reason for the doctor examining your conjunctivae if you go to the surgery complaining of tiredness and breathlessness), the corners of the mouth may be cracked and the nails may curl up at the edges and are what doctors call 'spoon-shaped'. In addition to these signs which can be observed, a patient with anaemia may complain of weakness, of shortness of breath, and of palpitations and giddiness on exertion. It is a straightforward condition to diagnose in the laboratory, and may even be diagnosed in a doctor's surgery with a simple blood test.

Pernicious anaemia is an anaemia which occurs classically in middle-aged, blue-eyed, white-haired people (we do not know why it is most common in these people) and is due to a deficiency of vitamin B_{12}. Our vitamin B_{12} needs are not very great, about one microgram per day, but if we cannot absorb it from our food, or, if once absorbed, we cannot utilize it, then the result is pernicious anaemia, with serious effects on the spine and nerves. Once diagnosed, a monthly injection of vitamin B_{12} can keep a person in normal good health.

The word 'anaemia' literally means 'without blood' and in all forms of anaemia, regardless of cause, there are characteristic changes in the blood, one of which interferes with the efficient transportation of oxygen and nearly always leads to weakness and shortness of breath. In very severe cases of anaemia, blood transfusion is necessary and a patient's health can be restored overnight by the administration of three or four pints of blood. However, this is rarely necessary and anaemia, in the main, is treated by tablets or injections. (For foods rich in iron and vitamins see p. 42.)

Angina Angina, or to give it its proper name, *angina pectoris*, meaning pain in the chest, is the severe pain which is symptomatic of too meagre a supply of oxygen to the heart muscle. This can occur because the blood-vessels supplying the heart muscle have become so narrow that they cannot carry sufficient blood, and therefore sufficient oxygen, to the heart muscle to cope with the normal conditions, or that they are only partially narrowed but cannot carry sufficient oxygen to the heart muscle when more oxygen than normal is needed, for instance during exercise, or after a meal. Most patients with angina have some degree of narrowing of the cardiac vessels.

The pain of angina is classically situated in the centre of the chest and radiates out to either shoulder and down either arm, but most commonly to the left. It may stop at the elbow or may go down to the wrist and fingertips. The pain may also radiate up from the centre of the chest, to the neck and into the jaw, and may resemble toothache. Again this may effect either side, but most commonly the left. Angina subsides when exercise or stress ceases. So a patient who suffers angina on walking will find that it goes if he stops, and a patient who suffers angina when he is anxious will find that it goes when he becomes calm.

There are some very effective treatments for angina, both old and new. One of the oldest is to slip a tablet of glyceryl trinitrate under the tongue. This substance is absorbed immediately into the blood-stream and will cause the cardiac vessels to dilate (open up) and allow more blood to reach the cardiac muscle, and with it more oxygen which relieves the pain of anoxia (lack of oxygen). Relief is almost instantaneous. Newer methods of treatment act in a more continuous way producing a dilation of the coronary vessels over a longer period and may pre-empt attacks of angina. Glyceryl trinitrate can and should be taken prophylactically. For instance, if an angina sufferer wishes to go out and do some gardening he can take a tablet prior to doing a bit of digging. Patients suffering from angina should always be under the care and regular attention of a doctor. (For helpful dietary advice and exercise programmes see pp. 65–7 and pp. 68–9.)

Anorexia Anorexia means loss of appetite. We lose our appetite under many normal situations, such as: anxiety, stress, depression, excitement or tiredness. Unless the precipitating cause is serious and the anorexia is long term, it does not need any treatment. Indeed most of us welcome it.

Anorexia is notoriously capricious in children. Some children can go for several days eating seemingly very little but nonetheless keep going and even thrive. This is because children need very much less food than we adults think they do and also because by eating in spurts they can very quickly make up for any deficiency that they incurred during a period when their appetite was lost.

In an otherwise healthy child who has a good appetite, loss of appetite, however, is one of the first symptoms of a serious illness and of an illness not necessarily related to the stomach. It can be the first symptom, for instance, of ear infections, of infectious disease or of appendicitis. Sudden loss of appetite in a child should always be taken seriously, especially if it is accompanied by vomiting and a high temperature.

In adults, similarly, loss of appetite can herald the onset of certain diseases which have nothing to do with the digestive tract. It is one of the first symptoms of infectious hepatitis and in many women it is one of the first symptoms of pregnancy. Appetite is nearly always lost with an infection of the kidney (pyelonephritis) which may be accompanied by vomiting. As in children, anorexia is one of the first symptoms of appendicitis.

Anorexia nervosa is a psychiatric condition mainly affecting young women which has become more commonly diagnosed in the last ten to fifteen years. It usually starts in a girl who is dieting to become slim. She becomes obsessive about the degree of slimness she wishes to obtain and equates not just slimness but thinness with beauty. She pursues the image of thinness with such perseverance that she is prepared to starve herself into an almost skeletal state.

One of the characteristics of anorexia is that patients frequently gorge themselves on food, then suffer immediate and retrospective remorse, force themselves to vomit and then undergo a period of severe deprivation. Severe cases may weigh less than six stones in weight and these patients require hospitalization and may even need intravenous feeding. They are always psychiatrically ill and there is frequently a background of psychiatric disturbance. Patients suffering from anorexia nervosa require a great deal of patience. Their recovery is slow and gradual and may take years; it depends heavily on psychoanalysis, group therapy, rehabilitation and parental support. The cause may lie deep in family relationships and many physicians recommend treating the family as well as the patient.

Appendicitis Appendicitis is inflammation of the appendix which is a small, elongated, balloon-like protuberance about two or three inches long situated at the beginning of the large bowel. The inflammation usually occurs after the narrow opening to the appendix has become blocked with a small piece of faeces. The normal mucus secretions of the bowel wall collect behind the blockage and this eventually causes the appendix to swell. The swollen tissues become infected, pus forms, and if not removed, the appendix will burst and liberate the pus into the abdominal cavity. This causes peritonitis and eventually an appendix abscess. Fortunately the symptoms of appendicitis are so classical and so easily recognized that most appendices are removed long before they reach a dangerous stage. The classical symptoms of appendicitis are: anorexia (loss of appetite); a moderately high temperature, around 100 °F. (37 °C.); pain which is first in the middle of the abdomen, around the umbilicus, and is colicky in nature (that means it comes and goes, reaches a crescendo and disappears). The pain then moves to the right side of the abdomen and the spot where the pain is present is tender to the touch.

An appendicectomy is usually a minor operation and the patient is walking, eating and drinking normally within twenty-four hours. There are no precautionary measures against appendicitis. Contrary to belief, it is rarely caused by pips that have been swallowed.

Arthritis There are many different forms of arthritis, from the harmless bony outgrowths on the last joint of the fingers seen in middle-aged women to the crippling rheumatoid arthritis which affects most of the joints of the hands and the feet and can also affect the knees, the elbows and the shoulders, and indeed several internal organs such as the lungs, the heart and the kidneys.

Arthritis simply means inflammation of the joints. The commonest form of arthritis is osteo-arthritis. This is really a part of the natural ageing process of the joints where the smooth, shiny, frictionless internal lining becomes rough and painful to move and the joint becomes swollen. The bony edges grow out and limit movement of the joint. Pain is worse as the day goes on when the joints have been used and are becoming tired. Osteo-arthritis affects mainly the weight-bearing joints, those which take the most strain, or joints which have been injured during life, such as the knees of rugger players. The hips, the knees and the feet are most commonly affected.

The final destruction of a joint by osteo-arthritis may be sufficient to make the joint useless. If this happens in the hip then the only remedy is to fit an artificial hip-joint. Surgical techniques are now so advanced and artificial hips are so beautifully designed that these operations are performed as a matter of routine and can give patients a new lease of life. They can allow a cripple, once confined to a wheelchair, to lead an active life again.

Rheumatoid arthritis is also a very painful disease of the joints but has a different pattern to osteo-arthritis. It does not affect the large, weight-bearing joints, it affects the smaller joints, like those of the hands and feet, and unlike osteo-arthritis it is most painful when the patient wakes up. Joints are very stiff at the beginning of the day with 'morning stiffness' which gradually wears off as the patient loosens up.

There are various forms of treatment for arthritis, the maxim of which is to combine sufficient exercise to keep the joints mobile with sufficient rest to soothe inflammation.

1 Heat treatment, such as warm baths and hot wax applications, is used to soothe and loosen up the joints.

2 Splints which keep the joints properly aligned are worn at night to prevent deformity of the joints and to rest them completely.

3 Various forms of physiotherapy and exercise programmes, various forms of walking aids, helpful gadgets around the house which make movements for arthritic hands easier, all contribute to making the arthritic's life more pleasant.

4 Symptomatic medical treatment relieves the pain and stiffness with anti-inflammatory/analgesic tablets, which can reduce inflammation and pain in the joints, and increases their mobility.

5 Surgical reconstruction of some joints which are destroyed can restore near-normal function.

A person with severe arthritis should always be in the regular care of a doctor.

Asthma The symptom common to all forms of asthma is wheezing. Wheezing is caused by the passage of air through narrow air passages. Whatever the cause of asthma the air passages are constricted, a situation worsened by the secretion of excessive thick mucus, and it is the air being breathed in and out through these narrowed tubes that causes the whistling sound of wheezing.

Because the air passages are contracted a great effort is required to get air in and out, and an asthmatic patient is in danger of becoming exhausted by the physical effort needed to breathe so treatment must be rapid. During an attack of asthma the patient becomes distressed, is unable to talk and the skin may gradually become blue because sufficient oxygen is not reaching the blood from the lungs.

Asthma can occur from childhood to senility. In infants it is a particularly difficult condition to treat as it often appears to be emotional in origin. The parents' job may be even harder if the child has infantile eczema as well. These two conditions often go together, but as a small bonus, children suffering from a combination of asthma and infantile eczema are unusually bright, intelligent, outgoing, very affectionate and rewarding to be with.

Infantile asthma and eczema may improve dramatically around the age of two and may disappear completely by the age of seven. The child may retain a sensitivity to develop bouts of wheezing and patches of eczema in their skin for the rest of their lives whenever they are under stress, e.g. exams, a severe illness, or a shock.

Asthma which persists through adolescence into adulthood is quite often allergic in origin. This means that the patient has become allergic to some foreign protein which is inhaled. The culprit is commonly house dust. Tests frequently show that the offending protein in house dust is a mite. When it is breathed in an allergic reaction in the muscles of the air passages causes them to constrict and an asthmatic attack ensues.

Even in cases where asthma is proven to be allergic in origin, emotional stress can bring on an attack. A chest infection can also be sufficient to cause an exacerbation of asthma. In these patients treatment with an antibiotic for the infection and with bronchodilators to dilate the air passages is necessary. A very severe attack of asthma always requires the emergency attention of a doctor because it may be necessary to treat the patient with a drug which requires injection. Difficulty with breathing *always* warrants calling your doctor.

Domestic treatment of an asthmatic should include:

1 Calling the doctor immediately if routine treatment, e.g. an inhaler, does not work.

2 Sit the patient up with three or four pillows.

3 Make sure the room is neither hot nor cold.

4 Undo any restrictive clothing.

5 Make sure the air is not too dry from central heating by keeping a kettle gently steaming in the room.

6 Never leave a child alone.

Another form of asthma which occurs in later life is bronchial-asthma. This type is a complication or a long-term result of chronic bronchitis and is extremely difficult to treat. Unfortunately, it is part of a chronic process of respiratory disease which ends up as crippling emphysema, when the elastic tissue of the lungs has broken down, preventing expansion and contraction and efficient ventilation. Patients suffering from emphysema are often respiratory cripples who become short of breath on taking a few steps and their lives are very seriously contained. (See also pp. 75–7.)

Athlete's foot Athlete's foot is an infection of the feet caused by a fungus. The fungus lives mainly between the clefts of the toes but the focus of the infection may be the toenails. Clearing the fungus from the skin is not sufficient if it is left lurking in the toenails from where it can re-infect the moist toe clefts. Some people suffer from athlete's foot and others do not, even though both have the fungus present on their feet. Whilst there is an underlying predisposition to develop fungous infections of the feet one of the most important factors is the presence of moisture. People with sweaty feet develop athlete's foot more readily than people with dry feet.

The diagnosis should always be proven by taking small scrapings of the skin from the webs of the toes, examining them under a microscope, seeing the fungus and recognizing it. Once identified it can be treated with certainty both with a specific cream (Whitfield's ointment) which will kill the fungus in the skin and tablets which are taken by mouth, enter the growing toenail and kill the fungus. Both these treatments are available on prescription. The tablets need to be taken for nine months to a year to allow the whole of the infected nail to grow out and be replaced by healthy nail.

Patent foot powders and patent treatments for athlete's foot will do little to eradicate the disease. The feet should be washed and dried at least twice a day and ideally the socks should be changed as often. Although athlete's foot is caused by an infectious agent it is not really a contagious disease in that the person picking up the fungus must have a predisposition to develop athlete's foot before the condition will take root. While the infection is active you should avoid swimming pools and wearing other people's shoes and socks. (See also **Feet complaints**.)

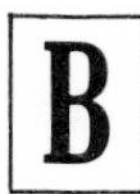

Back pain There are as many names for back pain as there are types of pain. Back pain is variously called lumbago, sciatica, fibrositis, slipped disc, all of which describe back pain that may be constant or sporadic, nagging or incapacitating, uncomfortable but allows you to soldier on, or excruciating so that you can hardly move at all, interferes very little with mobility or produces complete immobility.

The treatment of backache depends very much on whether it is an acute attack or a long-standing condition. Acute back pain (lumbago, sciatica) very often starts as a sudden pain in the loin while doing some fairly ordinary job, like gardening or sawing a piece of wood or having a game of golf. The pain is sufficient to prevent you from moving or standing upright, and although it usually starts in the loin it may extend into the groin, down into the buttock and the back of the thigh, right down the leg to the foot. Not only are movements affected, but sensation may also be diminished so that the skin of the leg and the foot tingles and feels numb. The usual cause of such acute pain is a strain of the ligaments or muscles, a slipped disc or a partially slipped disc.

Because most minor attacks recover in a fairly short time without any treatment, most doctors are loath to give medicine when rest would do. By rest your doctor means complete rest, and you should go to bed for four or five days and move your back as little as possible. It also helps to put a board under the mattress to support your back. Sometimes heat from a hot-water bottle will help, and massage by your husband or wife. The only other treatment would be analgesics to relieve the worst of the pain. Occasionally manipulation by a doctor or osteopath experienced in such manoeuvres can bring rapid and dramatic relief.

The treatment of chronic backache is more complex because it involves active treatment and prophylactic measures to prevent the back being strained in the future. Active measures would include rest, medication with analgesics or analgesic anti-inflammatory drugs, heat treatment, massage, manipulation by an expert, and exercises designed by your doctor or physiotherapist.

Exercising must be regular and done over a long period of time if the aim is to strengthen the spinal cord and abdominal muscles sufficiently to support the spinal column and improve the range of mobility. Exercise is one of the most important factors that can help in preventing a recurrent injury or strain which will exacerbate back pain. Exercises are also useful in helping to keep your weight down – an essential if you are a back-pain sufferer.

Prevention involves the alteration of habits and the modification of the way in which you do jobs; you should avoid standing and long periods of bending, and also use a back rest in your chair and car seat to keep the lower part of your back supported.

Occasionally these measures fail and then one must resort to wearing a spinal support in the form of a corset or belt. In a small number of cases, it is necessary to use surgical procedures to relieve the pain; the bones of the spinal column are fused during the operation, leaving a permanently stiff section of the back which rarely, however, interferes significantly with normal life. (See also section on posture, pp. 104–9.)

Barber's rash In adults, there is a condition caused by the bacterium, staphylococcus, which can affect the follicles in which the beard grows and a pustule forms around each hair. As the infection can get quite deeply into the hair follicle, this condition requires fairly radical treatment that may involve taking antibiotics by mouth, so you must consult your doctor about it. However, the same hygienic methods used for cleansing impetigo should be followed (see **Impetigo**).

Bed sores Bed sores are pressure ulcers. A pressure ulcer is caused by pressure on the skin which is sustained for a sufficient length of time to cut down its blood-supply. Oxygenation of the skin is diminished and its nourishment becomes deficient. Both of these factors contribute to loss of skin integrity on the pressure point. Once the surface of the skin is broken, continued pressure will lead ineluctably to an ulcer which will deepen and widen unless the pressure is relieved.

The appearance of a bed sore is a sign of nursing failure, and they are much more difficult to treat than to prevent.

The best treatment for bed sores is prevention, and with a patient who is immobile due to a stroke or an accident, those in charge of nursing care must make certain that the pressure points are resting on soft, pliable surfaces – an inflated seating ring is useful, as is a basket placed over the legs to hold off the weight of the bedclothes. Also the patient should be turned every hour so that no one area is exposed to long periods when it is carrying the whole weight of the body.

You can also take certain preventative measures which stimulate the circulation in the skin. This can be done very simply by rubbing or massaging the skin; and also by applying a liniment or ointment containing nicotinic acid which will dilate the blood-vessels of the skin, thereby promoting oxygenation and nourishment.

A bed sore may take months to heal over and requires assiduous and frequent treatment. No matter what you put on a bed sore, it will not heal if the pressure is not removed, so it is essential that the patient is moved constantly to keep pressure off the damaged area.

Home medical measures involve daily dressing of the wound. During the dressing, the wound is cleaned with antiseptic lotion and quite often an antiseptic vaseline gauze is put over the ulcer to prevent secondary infection and to help the edges heal inwards and upwards. Probably the most important aspect of healing bed sores is patience and persistence in the nursing.

Bilious attack As a child on Tyneside, I quite commonly heard that adults were indisposed due to 'bilious attacks'. This was a local term used to cover a multitude of conditions which in general presented the symptoms of headache, nausea and vomiting. Frequently the sufferers described themselves as being a bit 'liverish'.

These attacks would now be described as fatty indigestion, a symptom of gall-bladder disease; as abdominal migraine, where the abdominal symptoms are more dramatic than the headache; or as a hangover. Occasionally also the symptoms were probably referable to a mild attack of gastric flu and almost certainly to an exacerbation of a pre-existing peptic ulcer.

Whatever the cause, the home treatment for this group of abdominal symptoms is simple and can generally be applied as long as the temperature is normal and the symptoms do not prevail for longer than twelve or fifteen hours.

1 Take no food.

2 Take as much fluid as you can stomach.

3 Take analgesics which do not irritate the stomach, if you can take them, e.g. paracetamol.

4 Go to bed.

5 Go to sleep if you can.

6 Keep the room darkened.

7 If you have a mild sleeping pill in the house, take it. It is amazing how quickly abdominal symptoms subside if you can have four or five hours' sleep.

8 Make sure the room that you are in and the bed are warm.

Bites and stings

WASP AND BEE STINGS

1 Remove the sting from the skin if it is visible, with a pair of tweezers.

2 If you can do this shortly after the sting, apply strong negative pressure to the puncture by sucking hard, repeat this several times.

3 As wasp stings are alkali, the application of acid can sometimes help to neutralize the sting and relieve pain. A tablespoon of vinegar in a glass of water will serve as a very good bathing solution. A bee sting is acid so the application of sodium bicarbonate is a good remedy.

4 If the skin is hot and inflamed, apply a cooling fluid such as calamine lotion.

5 Do not be tempted to use local anaesthetic sprays or sprays that freeze the skin, their length of action is very short and the pain seems to be worse when it wears off.

6 If the skin looks particularly angry, apply a small quantity of antiseptic cream such as Savlon under a plaster.

7 If the face, lips or eyes begin to swell, go immediately to hospital as you may be allergic to the sting.

ANT BITES

Ants inject formic acid. This acid can be neutralized by applying an alkali and the common alkali around the house is soap or sodium bicarbonate.

1 If you can see the wound from the ant bite, suck it immediately to try to remove the formic acid.

2 Rub the spot with softened soap and let it dry.

3 Then use the procedures as outlined for a wasp sting if necessary.

SNAKE BITES
The bite of the commonest European snake, the adder, is painful and the part will usually swell up.

1 Calm and reassure the patient.

2 Do not cut or suck the wound.

3 Don't allow the patient to walk, but carry him to a convenient place to lie down.

4 Tie something like a handkerchief fairly firmly around the limb above the bite, sufficient to stop the blood flow in the veins, but not so tightly that the blood flow through the arteries is obstructed, so try and feel a pulse at the wrist or the ankle below the tourniquet.

5 If available wash the wound with soap and water, and then cover it with a piece of clean cloth.

6 Call your doctor or an ambulance whichever is the speediest.

Blackheads see **Acne.**

Blackouts see **Fainting.**

Bleeding A profusely bleeding wound or laceration is a medical emergency. The first step is to try to control the bleeding. This can best be done by pressing the edges of the wound together and holding firmly for at least five minutes. If bleeding persists, continue with hand pressure for a further ten minutes, then put a pad of clean material on top of the wound and keep it in place with a bandage. Go immediately to see your doctor or to the casualty department of the nearest hospital. If a lot of blood has been lost keep the patient lying down, with the head lower than the rest of the body and the feet tilted in the air, and call an ambulance. If the bleeding is not profuse, wash the wound in running water and then, while you protect it with a piece of clean material, wash the surrounding skin with soap and water, cover with a clean dressing and bandage. If there is a foreign body in the wound do not disturb it unless it is superficial and can easily be removed.

Blood This particular section deals with the appearance of blood in abnormal situations; for example, blood in the stools, or in the sputum. It must always be taken seriously and should prompt you to seek immediate medical help.

Blood in the motions or in urine or in vomit is not always bright red in colour, because it may undergo a chemical change which renders it a dark reddish brown colour or even black.

BLOOD IN THE MOTIONS Blood in the motions can be bright red which means that it has only recently entered the stools, and that the source is probably in the end of the bowel or the rectum. The causes, whilst troublesome, are normally not too serious and involve conditions like piles or an anal fissure, or even diverticulitis.

If bleeding occurs higher up in the bowel, such as in the stomach or duodenum, it will change colour during its passage through the bowel by the action of digestive enzymes and the stool will appear black. It is classically described as 'tarry'. The commonest cause of upper bowel bleeding is an ulcer, a gastric ulcer, or a duodenal ulcer. A black tarry stool (not the dark stool which results from taking liquorice medicine) always indicates a visit to your doctor because even a drop of blood lost from an ulcer, if it occurs over a long period of time, will make you anaemic. You have to have a diet, and active treatment to help heal the ulcer that is the cause of the bleeding.

A massive tarry stool or large amounts of fresh blood in the motion is a medical emergency. The patient should go to bed, lie flat, suck ice, be given no food and only water to drink, and an ambulance summoned.

BLOOD IN THE SPUTUM Blood appears in the sputum usually as reddish streaks and the commonest cause is explosive coughing. Coughing can rupture small blood-vessels at the back of the throat or in the larger bronchial tubes and only small amounts of blood are lost. Larger quantities are symptomatic of more serious conditions. In the old days they were suggestive of pulmonary tuberculosis, but now that this condition has been virtually eradicated the commonest cause of blood in the sputum is cancer of the lung.

BLOOD IN THE URINE Blood in the urine can also be fresh and red, or dark brown in colour. Fresh red blood usually is from the bladder or from the urethra which is the tube leading from the bladder to the outside. If it is red it means that it is produced just before or during the passage of the urine. If the blood is dark it means that it could have been in the bladder for some time and could have come from the kidney. By far the commonest cause of blood in the urine is an infection such as cystitis or venereal disease.

BLOOD IN THE VOMIT Blood can appear in the vomit for exactly the same reasons as it does in the sputum – the explosive movements of expelling the vomit may result in the breakage of small blood-vessels in the stomach and the oesophagus and small specks of bright red blood appear. Larger quantities nearly always arise from peptic ulcers and means that the ulcer has eroded a major artery which is bleeding profusely into the stomach. A patient suffering this amount of blood loss may become exsanguinated in a short time and must be regarded as a medical emergency. The patient will need an operation to stop the bleeding and a transfusion to replace lost blood.

Home first-aid treatment is the same as for massive haemorrhage in the stool.

INTER-MENSTRUAL BLEEDING It is quite normal for a woman to have spotting of blood from the vagina at the time of ovulation in the middle of the month, but bleeding at other times must be viewed with concern. Bleeding between periods or after intercourse should always take you to your doctor.

Boils A boil is a localized infection in the skin usually starting in a hair follicle caused by the bacterium staphylococcus.

It starts off as a small, red, tender lump, which enlarges and eventually 'points' with pus at the centre. The middle part usually softens, allowing the pus to escape. If it does not escape of its own accord the pustule may be pricked with a sterile needle and the pus can be gently eased out. A small pit will be left but normally fills in without leaving a scar. A large boil may contain a 'core' of semi-solid debris which cannot be squeezed out or easily removed. You should consult your doctor about how to treat this sequela of a boil as it may require special daily dressings.

Boils can be extremely painful if they occur in areas where the skin is stretched tightly over bone, such as the point of the chin or in the external ear canal. Any boil on the face should be treated rigorously so consult your doctor. They may also be troublesome in areas where hair grows, such as the back of the neck, and the armpit.

If boils recur, then you should go along to your doctor because you almost certainly have a focus of infection. This will act as a source of bacteria which are fed out on to the skin and cause the recurrent infections. The usual foci are chronic infections of the external auditory canal, chronic infections of the gums, teeth or eyes. Once the focus has been located, then it can be treated and eradicated. In the meantime, there are certain hygienic measures which you can take to cut down the number of bacteria on the skin.

You should pay particular attention to washing of the skin, and bathe every day, using an antiseptic soap. You should also use a mild antiseptic solution which you can obtain from your doctor (not a patent one) in your bathing and washing water. In addition you should wash your flannels and towels and nail brushes after each use, and if possible rinse them out in an antiseptic solution. You should take care not to allow anyone else in the house to use your toilet equipment.

Bronchitis Bronchitis means inflammation of the bronchi and is sometimes accompanied by a degree of tracheitis (inflammation of the trachea). The bronchi are the large air passages in the lungs. Inflammation of the bronchi for whatever cause results in some or all of the following symptoms: pain in the chest on taking in breath; pain in the chest on coughing; an excess of sputum which is coughed off the chest and the sputum may be creamy-white or yellow; possibly shortness of breath on exertion if severe; possibly a raised temperature if a secondary infection occurs.

The commonest cause of acute bronchitis is infection of the upper part of the airways by a virus such as the flu virus. The virus causes inflammation and secretion of increased quantities of mucus which are pushed up to the back of the throat by small hair-like strands lining the bronchi, then coughed into the mouth and spat out or swallowed. Rarely does the initial virus infection cause a serious illness unless it is a virulent virus, but quite often it weakens the bronchi sufficiently to pave the way for secondary invasion by bacteria and it is at this stage that the bronchitis may become a severe illness with a raised temperature, a severe cough and a lot of yellow infected sputum. If proper care and treatment is not given, bronchitis may progress to an infection of the lung, e.g. pneumonia.

If the bronchitis is not severe, the following home remedies will help:

1 Avoid sudden changes of temperature, such as those which occur going from a warm house into the cold outdoors.

2 Avoid hot dry air such as that found in heavily centrally heated rooms.

3 Try and stay in a room where the air is humidified, even if it is only by boiling a kettle in the room.

4 Try breathing an inhalant such as Friar's Balsam three times a day to soothe the irritated airways and ease the cough.

5 If you are coughing up yellow sputum, never use a cough suppressant medicine because it is part of the body's protective mechanism to get rid of that infection by coughing up the infected sputum.

6 Only if you have a dry irritant cough should you use a cough suppressant.

7 Treat a headache and aches and pains with simple analgesics, like paracetamol, that do not irritate the stomach.

If you have bronchitis which is accompanied by a high temperature you should always call your doctor because you are likely to need treatment with antibiotics. If you have recurrent attacks of bronchitis, you should have a chest X-ray. People who smoke always have an increased tendency to develop bronchitis and should bronchitis occur, it will be worse in a smoker than in a non-smoker.

If you have recurrent attacks of bronchitis, even if they are as far apart as each winter, and you are a smoker, you should stop smoking. You are on the slippery slope to chronic bronchitis and emphysema which will inevitably lead to cardiac problems and will be extremely disabling in later life.

Bunions A bunion is the enlargement and inflammation of the cushion of fluid which surrounds the joint of the big toe. The swelling of this fluid is the joint's response to being injured or strained over a long period of time.

The most common cause of bunions is ill-fitting shoes in early life. Bunions are infinitely more common in women than in men, and this is because of the wearing of high-heeled shoes or shoes which are badly fashioned, give little support to the foot and put a great deal of strain on the joint of the big toe. When wearing high-heeled shoes the whole weight of the body is transmitted through the single joint of the big toe.

Like most medical conditions it is better to prevent than to treat. Bunions can be prevented by wearing well-fitted, well-balanced shoes with heels that are not too high. The shape of the shoe should not be too pointed, and so avoid crushing the toes together, nor should the shape of the shoe press the big toe inwards from the longitudinal axis of the rest of the foot.

Once chronic inflammation in the joint of the big toe is set up it is very difficult to clear because the joint is irritated with every step that we take. The healing of an early bunion, or to use its proper medical term bursitis, necessitates complete rest for several weeks and most people are not prepared to do this.

Having developed a large bunion, the only satisfactory treatment is surgery, and this involves cutting away the chronically inflamed sac of fluid which surrounds the joint and then fixing the joint so that it is permanently stiff. The operation results in a total relief of pain and a slight disability in walking. It also involves being in bed for six weeks after the operation and not taking any weight on the feet. For most people it is difficult to fit such a long period of rest into their normal lives.

Burns Burns vary in severity from a minor injury in the kitchen which causes a blister, and which one often ignores, to a severe localized burn or scald which kills all the layers of the skin and can only be repaired by a skin graft. The most serious burns involve large areas of the body and endanger the patient's life. The following comments apply only to those burns which are not serious enough to require expert medical attention and are largely confined to 'first-degree burns' which produce a reddening or blistering of the skin over small areas.

1 Keep the burnt part as cold as possible for as long as possible. Simply running a burnt hand under a cold tap for several minutes will diminish the amount of damage that is done to the skin, for the following reasons. If you lower the temperature of the skin, the rate of metabolism of the skin is also lowered. This means that the nutritional needs of the skin are temporarily diminished and the skin cells can live with a lower concentration of oxygen and nutrients. So cooling of a burnt part of the body can stop the cells from dying and can prevent damage to the skin. Placing ice on the burnt area is probably even better. When the part becomes very cool and painful due to exposure to cold remove it for a few seconds from the cold and then re-apply the cold. The longer you can go on doing this, the less the damage will be. We have avoided many a blister and many a bad burn in our family by following this very simple first-aid manoeuvre.

2 The pain from a minor burn will probably last for three or four hours and there is no harm in giving a child an analgesic to see them over this period. Don't be tempted to use local anaesthetic sprays: application to the skin can cause skin allergies which can become serious if you have to go to the dentist and have a local anaesthetic injection.

3 If the integrity of the skin has been broken apply a simple antiseptic cream such as Savlon.

4 If a blister appears, don't burst it immediately – it is nature's own protective pad. Cover it with a plaster.

5 If the blister persists, prick it with a needle sterilized by wafting it in a flame for about a minute.

6 Once the blister has been pricked, cover with a plaster which has been smeared with a small quantity of antiseptic cream.

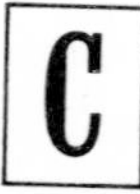

Cardiac arrest see **Kiss of life.**

Catarrh I and, I am sure, most doctors are uncertain as to what patients mean when they say they are suffering from catarrh. Catarrh is not a word used by doctors. What I understand patients mean by catarrh is a thick tenacious post-nasal drip running down the back of the throat which is fairly common during or after a cold, and can be a residual symptom after an attack of sinusitis or may be persistent in chronic sinusitis. If the catarrh is infected, it usually has a very unpleasant taste. If this is the nature of your catarrh, then treatment with antibiotics is almost certainly indicated and you should consult your doctor.

Simple catarrh which is part of a cold need not be treated. It is a short-term self-limiting condition, and will disappear when the cold has gone. Catarrh which is part of sinusitis should be viewed in the same way. It will disappear when the sinusitis is treated with antibiotics and is cleared. If, however, you suffer from chronic catarrh due to chronic sinusitis, then the sinusitis should be confirmed with X-rays. If your doctor thinks it is appropriate, you should have long-term treatment with antibiotics. The complete eradication of a chronic infection in the sinuses usually requires antibiotic treatment for six weeks at least. Sinus wash-outs may be considered for recalcitrant cases.

Please avoid using the following treatments; they will produce only transient relief of symptoms or may even make them worse in the long run: the chronic use of nose drops whatever they contain; the use of nose drops which contain such substances as ephedrine or isoprenaline – these nose drops should only be given under medical supervision because the long-term use of such substances can result in damage to the lining of the nose and sinuses; use of nasal sprays which are not prescribed by your doctor as these can often worsen the irritation and therefore produce more catarrh rather than curing it.

Chilblains Chilblains are a condition of the skin due to exposure to cold. First there is a constriction of the small blood-vessels in the skin. When the skin is warmed up, the blood-vessels dilate and this produces an itchiness in the skin which if scratched can result in a lumpy, irritable inflamed patch in the affected part of the skin. The blood-vessels may over-compensate when warmed and stay dilated for longer than normal which makes the chilblain persistently itchy.

Some people have a predisposition to develop chilblains because their skin is more sensitive to the effect of cold than others. These people should take precautions to make sure their skin does not become exposed to cold. For people with poor circulation, this is often difficult and involves wearing several layers of 'thermal' clothing, which fortunately is much more common than it used to be. Indeed with the sensible fashion of boots and leg-warmers in cold weather, chilblains are much rarer than they used to be.

The application of patent medicines will do little to help chilblains, particularly if one does not take precautions to prevent the skin from being exposed to cold. The aim should be to maintain the temperature of the skin as constant as possible by protecting it from the cold, thereby preventing the alternate constriction and dilation of the blood-vessels in the skin. Wear warm socks, boots and thermal in-soles.

Choking Each year many people die in public places such as restaurants from choking without anyone coming to their aid.

1 If an infant or small child is choking, take hold of them by the ankles and hold upside down, and then strike them sharply between the shoulder blades. It is worth repeating this a couple of times to dislodge the material which is causing choking.

2 If an older child is choking, lay them face down over your knee with the head dangling over the side of your legs, then give them three or four sharp blows between the shoulder blades.

3 If an adult is choking, try three or four sharp blows between the shoulders, which should bring the material up to the back of the throat, then remove the material from the throat. If they don't breathe, try the kiss of life (see pp. 178–9).

If all these methods fail, the patient is turning blue, there is no skilled help available, and the emergency is therefore dire, you should try to perform a tracheotomy if there is a sharp-bladed instrument available. Your courage may save a life. Take heart – there are few crucial structures between the skin and the windpipe.

1 Lay the patient on his back.

2 Put your finger in the notch at the top of the breast bone and press down firmly.

3 You should be able to feel the trachea or main wind pipe which is identifiable by the rings of stiff cartilage which run around it.

4 Hold the blade vertically over this point of the skin and push it straight downwards towards the floor for about ¾ in.

5 As the blade enters the trachea you will hear a hiss as air rushes into the lungs.

6 Turn the blade of the knife through 90° so that the hole in the trachea is left open and hold it open until help arrives and a tube can be inserted.

Cold The common cold is caused by a virus which affects the lining of the throat, the nose, the eyes and sometimes the air passages. There is no known cure. Your doctor can provide you with no better treatment than you yourself can, so there is no point in visiting him with a common cold unless you are suffering from some underlying medical condition and he has asked you to report to him the advent of a cold.

The common cold is one of the few conditions where patent medicines serve a really useful purpose and I would suggest that you try the many varieties that are offered and use the one which brings you most relief.

Cold sores Cold sores are caused by a virus which is closely related to the virus of chickenpox. It lies dormant in the skin most of the time. Whilst the virus is dormant there are no symptoms, but once it becomes active, a cold sore appears. The virus is made active when the skin is heated up. As this occurs most frequently when you have a temperature, i.e. a 'cold', these classical blisters and scabs of cold sores were so named. However, people who suffer from cold sores will tell you there are many other exacerbating factors than the common cold which would include exposure to the sun, becoming very excited and heated, being in a very hot atmosphere, and ovulation (at ovulation the body temperature may increase as much as one degree and cold sore sufferers quite often have an outbreak of blisters at the middle of the month when ovulation occurs).

Cold sores frequently affect the face and are most common in a band between the chin and the eyes. They are transmitted from one person to another by kissing and if a mother suffers from cold sores, most of her children probably will too, not to mention her husband. Cold sores around the eyes and those involving the eyes, need urgent medical attention, because if blisters occur on the surface of the eye they may result in a scar and affect eyesight.

There is no magic remedy in the treatment of cold sores and there is very little that a doctor can prescribe to speed up the healing of a cold sore. Their natural history, regardless of any medication, is nearly always ten to fourteen days from the appearance of the blisters to complete healing.

Cold sores nearly always begin with a tingling sensation in the skin. This is the only time that treatment can make any difference to the development of a cold sore. There is an ointment containing a chemical called idoxuridine (available on prescription), and which if applied as soon as these early symptoms appear and re-applied at intervals of half an hour, may abort the appearance of the cold sore in about half the patients who use it. Once the sore has got to the blister stage there is nothing you can do about it other than try to ease the discomfort, and opinion is divided on how best to do this. Some people say it is best to keep it dry with astringent lotion such as surgical spirit. Others say it is best to keep it soft with greasy ointments such as vaseline. All I can say is to take your pick. Nothing will make very much difference.

Colic Colic is a pain which is caused by the spasmodic contractions of any smooth muscle. Smooth muscle is the kind that we have in our internal organs such as the bladder, the intestine, stomach and the womb. Smooth muscle is contracting and relaxing much of the time causing no pain at all. Colicky pain occurs when the smooth muscle goes into a very tight prolonged contraction to overcome a blockage.

All colicky pain is the same regardless of what sort of muscle is affected and what the cause is. The pain has the following classical features: it comes and goes in waves, it starts gradually, becomes more severe, builds to a crescendo and then dies away; at its peak it may be excruciating; it disappears completely once the blockage is overcome.

The commonest form of colic is that which is caused by spasmodic contraction of the bowel and is an everyday occurrence in that the pain of wind is caused by the bowel going into spasm while attempting to move on a bubble of gas.

The most painful form of colic is renal colic and this is due to spasm of the ureter (the tube which conducts urine from the kidney to the bladder). Blockage of the ureter is nearly always caused by a kidney stone which has become dislodged from the kidney and has been carried into the ureter. Sufferers of renal colic describe it as the worst pain they have ever experienced, and it continues until the spasmodic contractions of the ureter push the stone down into the bladder.

Very severe colic of any kind which causes the patient to cry out or sweat profusely and which continues for longer than an hour, warrants summoning the doctor. For other forms of colic, a hot-water bottle and a mild analgesic are the best treatment as it will almost certainly pass off of its own accord.

Dysmenorrhoea or painful periods can be caused by spasmodic contractions of the uterine muscle. Very often there is a psychological aspect to this pain but sufferers claim it is severe enough to take them to bed. Many medical authorities suggest that this is entirely the wrong treatment and dysmenorrhoea sufferers would do a lot better taking a brisk walk and a mild analgesic. Dysmenorrhoea is also self-limiting in that the pain usually subsides when menstrual flow is established. Simple analgesics do help and there is a newer group of drugs which are thought to relieve specifically the uterine colic of dysmenorrhoea.

Colitis Colitis means inflammation of the colon. It occurs most commonly in any mild infection of the bowel by a non-virulent virus. This form of colitis therefore does not warrant any specific treatment.

This mild form of colitis nearly always results in some diarrhoea and symptomatic treatment would be taking a mixture of kaolin and morphine. This can be bought at any chemist and will dry up the stools. Mild analgesics can be taken if the discomfort is sufficient.

Even mild colitis cannot be treated so lightly in small infants however, because they quickly become dehydrated and the necessity to rehydrate them can be very urgent in a very short time. You should always call your doctor if your child has prolonged diarrhoea with abdominal pain and particularly if he or she is vomiting and has a temperature. Almost all other forms of colitis in children and prolonged colitis in adults (more than forty-eight hours) require medical care and you should seek it from your doctor.

Concussion Concussion is loss of consciousness due to a blow on the head. After such a blow the blood-vessels of the brain contract so that the brain cells receive an inadequate supply of blood. As a result they cannot function properly and unconsciousness may ensue. The length of unconsciousness is largely dependent on the degree of damage to the brain. Sometimes it may be bruised and there may even be small haemorrhages within the brain itself. In this case, concussion may last days, weeks or even months. At the other end of the scale, the disturbance of consciousness may be very slight, restricted only to dizziness.

Home treatment would involve the patient being kept in bed in a dark, quiet room, without pillows so that the head is low. When consciousness returns the head may be gradually raised and the patient should stay in bed for three or four days if the concussion has been short, and for at least a fortnight if the concussion has lasted a week or more. People who suffer concussion may notice that they are slightly more irritable than usual and that they are unable to concentrate for a few weeks after their accident.

Anyone who suffers a severe blow to the head or has concussion must have a skull X-ray as soon as possible.

Conjunctivitis Conjunctivitis is inflammation of the conjunctiva, the outermost covering of the eye. The eye has a gritty feeling and the discomfort may be a soreness or smarting sensation. The eye is nearly always red and waters quite a lot, and sufferers tend to avoid bright light.

Conjunctivitis can be caused by chemical or physical agents. Chemical agents would be irritant gases or acids, physical agents would be dust or grit and extremes of heat or cold. Conjunctivitis can be viral or bacterial in origin.

Any home treatment for conjunctivitis should be simple and short and if the condition does not respond, then medical help should be sought immediately. Do not use any patent eye drops if you have a red, sore, watering eye. The best thing that you can use is a solution of one teaspoonful of salt per pint of warm water as an eye wash, and repeat this three or four times a day. If the soreness and redness does not improve within a few hours, then your conjunctivitis is going to need therapy which can only be prescribed by a doctor, so contact him immediately.

Constipation Constipation can be more in our minds than in our bowels. The British nation as a whole is probably more fixated about bowel regularity than with any other aspect of health. British mothers certainly are, and many of us bear the scars of the old-fashioned and now well-outdated potty-training routines where babies' bowels had to conform to the regularity of their mother's expectations. A child or adult who is taking a balanced diet which contains fresh fruit, green vegetables and a fair degree of roughage in the form of wholemeal bread or bran, should have no problems with constipation whether or not they have a bowel movement every day. Not everyone is given to having a bowel movement every day and a person who only passes a stool twice a week is not necessarily constipated; the frequency of their bowel motions still falls within the limit of what doctors would consider normal, and no treatment is required.

By far the best treatment for a sluggish bowel is to increase the amount of roughage in the diet, with fibrous fruit and vegetables. The old-fashioned remedy of a few stewed prunes every morning for breakfast, or some figs, fresh or dried, not necessarily a syrup, is a good substitute. Certainly in children one should avoid the use of purgatives at all costs.

In adults, constipation responds best to a revision of bowel habit. The bowel is really a very efficient machine. As soon as food is taken and enters the stomach, the bowel responds with what is known as the gastro-colic reflex or 'the call to stool', that is, the bowel tells the brain that it wishes to empty itself. Most of us with busy lives have been ignoring the call to stool for so long that the bowel has ceased to give it. What we have to do is to encourage the bowel to restart sending us messages and to respond to them. If we do, we will find that our bowels regulate themselves without further help.

Hard, dry stools are usually hard and dry because the call to stool has been ignored and all the water has been absorbed from the stool while it has been waiting in the rectum. The way to correct this fault is to obey the call to stool and to take more fluid in the diet. As bran and cellulose hold water in the stool, increasing the amount of fibre and bran in the diet will also help to soften the stool. Regular use of patent purgatives only makes the bowel lazier.

Convulsions Febrile convulsions in children are a fairly common occurrence as they are the expression of the general way brain cells react to a high body temperature. A child's tendency to respond to a fever with convulsions varies: some do and some don't. Children may also occasionally have a convulsion after being given their immunization injections. In whatever situation it occurs you must inform your doctor.

The appearance of convulsions in a sick child is not sufficient to label him as an epileptic. In children and adults, epileptic convulsions are due to abnormal brain activity. It is important to make a correct diagnosis because epilepsy is an eminently treatable condition and sufferers can lead a perfectly normal life with the correct medication.

An epileptic fit classically has a sudden onset when the patient falls to the ground, the jaws are usually clenched and breathing becomes noisy and laboured. Many of the body muscles jerk or become rigid and the patient may urinate or defecate because bladder and bowel control may be lost. When the muscle jerking involves the muscles of the jaw, the saliva may become bubbly and the patient is said to be 'frothing at the mouth'.

Whilst epilepsy is the commonest cause of a convulsion in adults, a convulsion may occur whenever the brain is irritated, such as in meningitis or a stroke, in kidney failure or liver failure, and occasionally even in heat stroke when the body temperature-regulating mechanism is lost and the body temperature may rise steeply.

Home treatment for a convulsion is a matter of making sure that the person injures himself as little as possible:

1 Move any obstacles away from them.

2 Loosen any tight clothing around the neck to make sure that they can breathe freely.

3 If they are champing their jaws or their teeth are clenched, you should try to wedge a handkerchief or paper between the teeth so that the clamping motions do not damage the tongue.

After the fit, keep the person lying down and they may fall asleep for several hours. On waking they may remember nothing, but complain of aches and pains due to the muscle spasms.

Home treatment for a child with a febrile convulsion would be to try to lower his temperature. Once the convulsion is over you would:

1 Inform your doctor.

2 Sponge the child down in bed with tepid water.

3 Use a fan to blow cool air over him.

4 Cover him with only a light sheet.

5 Give him the appropriate dose of soluble aspirin which is a very effective anti-pyrexial agent.

Cough A cough is either productive or non-productive: a productive cough produces sputum; a non-productive cough produces nothing.

A productive cough that is getting rid of sputum from the chest be it infected or not, is a useful cough and therefore should not be suppressed. Indeed, it should be encouraged with expectorant medicines that help to loosen the mucus and encourage coughing debris out of the lungs. On no account use a suppressant cough medicine for a productive cough.

A non-productive cough, however, which is nothing more than an irritant and prevents sleep, and makes the throat and chest sore, can be suppressed with safety. The most efficient cough suppressant which acts on the cough centre in the brain is codeine and many proprietary codeine cough mixtures are available from the chemist. It is important not to exceed the stated dose as codeine has serious side effects. One of the less serious is constipation. If you have to take a cough suppressant medicine for more than twenty-four hours, you can expect mild constipation. Your bowel action will return to normal within a couple of days.

The cough of whooping cough with the characteristic whoop at the end may come in prolonged paroxysms and eventually end with the child vomiting. Whooping cough is a serious condition, not just because it is contagious, but because it may leave the lungs permanently damaged. Whooping cough always warrants a call to your doctor.

Another cough which should always be treated seriously is one which appears out of the blue and is persistent. The reason for treating it seriously is that it may be due to stimulation of the nerve which supplies the back of the throat and therefore may be due to dental trouble or ear trouble which will need treating quite independently of the cough.

If your cough causes severe pain in the centre of your chest or anywhere around the sides or the lower part of the chest, you should tell your doctor because it may be the first symptom of tracheitis (inflammation of the main airway) or of pleurisy. And though you may have neither of these conditions, you should alert your doctor.

Cramp Cramp is a pain caused by a spasm of skeletal muscle. Skeletal muscles are those which are attached to bones and joints and which are responsible for the movement of our limbs and the various parts of our body.

Muscles can go into cramp for a variety of reasons, but most of these are referable to a lack of oxygen, or a change in the electrical charge on the muscle fibre. Cramp that we get when we go swimming after a meal is due to the former because most of the blood has been diverted to the stomach to deal with digestion, leaving relatively little for the muscles that work during swimming.

A change in the electrical charge on the muscle is responsible for the kind of cramp that comes on for no reason at all, usually at night. It is thought that this type of cramp is due to an alteration in the concentration of sodium ions on the surface of the muscle fibre, and one of the forms of treatment that works very well is half a teaspoonful of salt dissolved in a glass of water taken just before going to bed. This form of treatment would not be indicated in patients who are suffering from any form of heart disease, but it is a good treatment to try if you are otherwise perfectly healthy.

Croup For the treatment of croup see *Miriam Stoppard's Book of Babycare*.

Cystitis Cystitis means inflammation of the lining of the bladder and when this occurs, the muscle in the wall of the bladder becomes irritated and goes into spasm and causes severe pain. The pain of cystitis, whilst it may be fairly constant, is worse when the bladder empties. When this happens, it contracts down from a balloon shape into a small ball, and the muscles tighten up to expel the last drop of urine. This distortion of the inflamed lining causes pain. Pain at the end of passing urine in the presence of cystitis can be absolutely awful.

The inflamed lining of the bladder also becomes hypersensitive to the presence of urine, so if a little urine collects in the bladder the lining is stretched. This stretching is sufficient to set off contractions in the irritable muscle, bringing on the desire to pass urine. Someone suffering from cystitis may be constantly running to the lavatory to pass only a few drops of urine. If the inflammation is very severe, the urine may be blood-stained. The pain from cystitis may not be confined to the lower pelvis but may radiate through to the back and up into the loins. If this occurs and the loins become tender and in addition you get a high temperature, this probably means that an infection has ascended from the bladder to the kidneys. This is a very serious condition called pyelonephritis and needs urgent treatment by your doctor.

The cause of cystitis can be infective or mechanical. Infections need to be treated with antibiotics and for that you need to visit your doctor. Take along a specimen of urine so he can examine it on the spot and save time in prescribing treatment.

Mechanical types of cystitis have been recognized only recently, and are blamed on the wearing of tights, motor-cycle riding, etc. During the war there was a land army girl's cystitis which was due to the bumping the girls received while driving tractors. If the mechanical forms are not associated with infection, then no more treatment is needed other than removing the mechanical irritation and drinking copious quantities of water to keep the inflamed lining of the bladder constantly washed out. Another simple home remedy is to add half a teaspoonful of sodium bicarbonate to a glass of water and drink that three or four times a day. This makes the urine alkaline and helps to suppress the growth of bacteria in urine. Sometimes muscle-relaxant drugs are helpful and your doctor will advise you if you need them.

If you have severe infected cystitis you must obtain treatment from your doctor. It will be helped in any event by the above two suggestions of drinking lots of fluid and taking bicarbonate of soda in water three or four times a day. Much helpful information is available from the Cystitis Society, U & I Club, 9e Compton Road, London, N1.

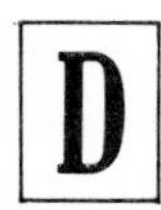

Dandruff Dandruff is the piling up of dead skin cells which, if it were not for the hair, would be shed freely without us even noticing. Some people suffer from it because their skin sheds scales faster than those of us who do not. The remedy is not to use specially formulated anti-dandruff shampoos containing 'anti-dandruff chemicals'. These chemicals are sometimes an irritant to the scalp, and the more often they are used, in the mistaken belief that the more often you use a medicine the more quickly you will be cured, the more irritating they are. The correct treatment procedure is quite the opposite: *use a mild shampoo, and underwash the hair*. Here are some tips for dandruff sufferers:

1 Never brush the hair vigorously as this only stimulates the scalp to produce more scales.

2 Never massage the scalp as this does the same as vigorous brushing.

3 Don't use anti-dandruff shampoos more frequently than once a fortnight. Anything which irritates the scalp only stimulates it to produce more scales and therefore worsens the dandruff rather than helps it.

4 Use the mildest shampoo you can get hold of, for example a baby shampoo, when you wash your hair.

5 Wash your hair fairly often, say every two or three days.

6 The routine to follow when washing your hair is to take a teaspoonful of shampoo, dissolve it in a glass of warm water, wet your hair, pour the glass over the head, and gently with your fingertips massage the shampoo into a mild lather. Never rub, never scrub, never scratch. Leave the shampoo in contact with the hair for about two minutes and then rinse off. Don't shampoo twice.

If your dandruff is really severe it may not be dandruff at all. It may be a seborrhoeic dermatitis or psoriasis. In either case you require specialist treatment from a dermatologist, so ask your general practitioner if he feels that referral to a dermatologist would be useful.

Diarrhoea Diarrhoea is the bowel's response to irritation. When the lining of the bowel is irritated by whatever cause, it responds by doing two things: by producing more mucus than normal which contributes to a loose, slimy stool; and by speeding up the waves of contraction, which normally pass down the bowel rather slowly and regularly. They begin to move very frequently and irregularly, resulting in intestinal hurry.

Both of these things produce abdominal pain which may be colicky (see **Colic**) and a thin, watery stool. It is mainly intestinal hurry which is responsible for this latter symptom. Under normal conditions, water is gradually absorbed as the stool is moving through the bowel, and the stool gradually thickens and becomes more bulky. When the stool is 'hurried' through the colon, there is not time for the water to be absorbed and the stool has a thin, watery consistency.

The dangers of diarrhoea in young patients are discussed under **Colitis**. In adults diarrhoea can be harmful if it is severe and prolonged, as it is in some serious infections like typhoid and cholera, when large quantities of fluids and important minerals are lost in a very short time.

Diarrhoea needs to be treated according to its severity and cause. The diarrhoea that we all occasionally suffer due to nerves or anxiety needs no treatment at all because the anxiety and nervousness is usually short lived and therefore limits the length of the diarrhoea attack.

The sort of diarrhoea brought on by a change of diet or water rarely needs medical treatment because our bodies adjust to these changes fairly quickly.

Viral forms of diarrhoea, unless the virus is a very virulent one, also require only mild or symptomatic treatment, such as:

1 Eschewing all solid food.

2 Taking plenty of fluids.

3 Taking a mild 'closing' medicine such as kaolin and morphine, available from any chemist.

4 A mild analgesic if the abdominal discomfort is unpleasant.

5 Gradually introducing a bland diet as the diarrhoea subsides.

You should seek medical help if your diarrhoea is any more severe than that described because it will need specific medical treatment which can only be obtained from a doctor. If you experience diarrhoea which alternates with constipation you should discuss the change of bowel habit with your doctor who will investigate it to see if it has any serious cause.

Discharge, Vaginal For most days of the month the majority of women have a certain amount of vaginal discharge which is entirely normal. In the first half of the month, vaginal discharge tends to be a fairly thin and runny colourless mucus, which becomes quite profuse in quantity at the time of ovulation (fourteen days after the first day of the last period). Then in the second part of the month the discharge alters in character and becomes a more sticky, tenacious, thicker, opaque discharge. Both of these discharges are quite normal, and when they dry, tend to be rather creamy yellowish in colour.

If you are concerned as to whether you have an *abnormal* vaginal discharge, there are two fairly simple tests that will help you decide:

1 The first is smell. A discharge due to an infection always has an unpleasant smell. If your vaginal discharge does not have an unpleasant smell it is very unlikely that it is abnormal.

2 The second is irritation. Normal vaginal discharge does not irritate the genital parts, whereas an abnormal discharge associated with infection invariably does.

So in summary, if there is no bad smell and no irritation, it is unlikely that your vaginal discharge is anything to worry about.

If you have a vaginal discharge with either unpleasant characteristic, consult your doctor immediately because there is nothing that you can do to treat it. It usually needs rigorous antibiotic therapy to eliminate it. In particular, don't feel that you can get rid of a discharge by putting antiseptic fluids in your bath water. This can actually be harmful to you and create an irritation not just of the vagina, but also of the urethra, and even lead to cystitis. Don't ever be tempted to put antiseptics in your bath water as a prophylaxis against contracting an infection be it of skin or vagina, unless instructed to do so by your doctor. (See also **Venereal diseases**.)

Diverticulosis/Diverticulitis The condition of diverticulosis which is symptomless, always precedes the condition of diverticulitis which is inflammation in small diverticula in the lower bowel. These diverticula are small balloonings of the lining of the large bowel through weak spots in the muscular wall. This occurs in all of us to some extent as we get older and the wall of the bowel loses its strength, but research over the last five or ten years has shown that diverticulosis is far more common amongst races whose diet is low in fibre and rich in synthetic foods. In fact, diverticulosis and diverticulitis are virtually unknown in primitive communities where the diet contains a large amount of roughage. These small pouches can be shown up quite clearly on an X-ray film if a barium enema is performed, and in a severe case one may see twenty or thirty fairly large diverticula of the colon.

It is only a matter of time before these diverticula become inflamed and when they do, we have the condition of diverticulitis with the classical symptoms that have been grouped together to give 'left-sided appendicitis'. The symptoms include pain on the left side of the abdomen, tenderness down in the left groin and fever. When the condition becomes chronic it may result in constipation or irregular bowel actions and pain on evacuation of the bowels, which often warrants treatment with special antibiotics from your doctor. Nonetheless there are certain steps that you can take to minimize the trouble that your condition will give you:

1 Try to improve the quality of your diet and increase the quantity of fibre that you eat.

2 Make sure that you drink plenty of fluid to keep the stool fairly soft; never disobey the call to stool and make sure that you evacuate your bowel whenever you feel the reflex to do so.

3 Avoid foods that may irritate the bowel such as onions or peas and highly spiced foods like curry.

Best of all, avoid diverticulosis in the first place by making sure that your diet contains sufficient fibre and roughage.

Dizziness The causes of dizziness are legion and beyond the scope of this book. If you have attacks you must see your doctor for a full investigation of your condition. The things which you can do to help yourself are few and simple:

1 If you feel an attack coming on, sit down immediately.

2 Put your head between your knees, if possible.

3 Lie down completely flat, if possible.

4 Lie down flat with your head lower than the rest of your body, if possible.

5 Get up very slowly when the sensation of dizziness has passed.

6 Do not drive a car.

Drowning The most important thing is to get air into the lungs as soon as possible. As long as you have a firm footing, start the kiss of life (see pp. 178–9) while still in the water.

Dysmenorrhea see **Colic.**

Dyspepsia Dyspepsia literally means a malfunctioning digestive system, but we interpret it to mean 'stomach trouble' and indigestion in particular.

If half a dozen people were asked to describe indigestion, we would have half a dozen different descriptions. But in general, indigestion means discomfort in the stomach a short time after taking food, possibly accompanied by a sensation of acidity even with regurgitation of acid fluid into the mouth, plus heartburn – a burning sensation behind the breastbone. People who complain of indigestion often use the words 'acid indigestion' or 'fatty indigestion' meaning that the stomach feels acid after food or that their indigestion is associated with fatty foods.

If indigestion is not associated with over-indulgence, it is usually due to an excessive secretion of acid in the stomach. All of us are born with the same number of acid-secreting cells in the stomach. We all vary, however, in the amount of acid which each of these cells is capable of secreting. Those of us who secrete the most may end up with a duodenal ulcer, those of us who secrete normal quantities will have no symptoms at all, and those people in between may occasionally suffer from various forms of acid indigestion.

Persistent acid indigestion should always be investigated by your doctor, but there are certain things that you can do to help yourself.

1 Never eat a very large meal.

2 Try to eat small meals frequently:

3 Try to avoid very rich or fatty foods.

4 If you get a touch of indigestion resort first to natural treatments rather than synthetic ones; by natural, I mean a glass of milk. A synthetic treatment would be an antacid mixture or tablet, or bicarbonate of soda.

5 Never over-indulge in antacid remedies. Sodium bicarbonate, for instance, taken in large quantities by the mouth, can seriously damage the body's acid/alkali balance.

6 Never let the stomach get really empty of food. It is better to take a cup of tea and a biscuit between meals than to wait until you get home for a full meal. This is because there is nothing to mop up the acid in an empty stomach. Conversely, over-eating encourages the secretion of excessive amounts of acid.

7 Keep a drink and a biscuit on your bedside table in case you wake with indigestion.

8 If you wake at night with indigestion, sleep propped up with several pillows.

(See also **Gallstones**.)

Duodenal ulcer see **Peptic ulcer**.

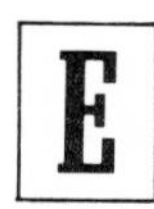

Earache Earache can be due to: causes referable to the ear; causes not referable to the ear. In the first group, pain arises from inflammation of the external ear canal, of the middle ear, or complications of middle-ear infections. Whatever the cause, in whichever situation, proper treatment can only be obtained from your doctor, so you must consult him immediately.

Causes of earache which are not directly associated with the ears include: a faulty jaw joint which may slip out of true when the mouth is opened wide; impacted lower molars; infected undescended wisdom teeth; tonsillitis; swollen glands in the neck from tonsillitis or other throat infections; neuralgia of the face or tongue.

Earache warrants only one first-aid measure that you yourself can take and that is the use of analgesics. Remember:

1 Don't wash out the ears.

2 Don't put ear drops into the ears.

3 Don't put warm oil into the ears.

4 Don't put anything hard like a hairpin into the external ear canal.

5 Don't push a cotton bud into the external ear.

If a foreign body gets into the ear such as a bead or a pea, do not try to remove it yourself, and do not poke anything into the external canal, because you may push the object further down the canal and rupture the ear drum. Take the person to the nearest hospital casualty department.

Ears, Ringing in In children the commonest cause of ringing in the ears is wax in the external canal which is not a serious condition and can be treated at your doctor's surgery by syringing.

In adults, the commonest cause of ringing in the ear is Menière's disease which is an abnormality of the balance organ of the inner ear and is thought to be a disturbance of water metabolism. Attacks of profound dizziness, vertigo, nausea, vomiting and unsteady gait can be so severe that they make the patient fall down. If prolonged they are incapacitating because of the vomiting and the patient may be confined to bed because of the ataxia (unsteady gait). Menière's disease is amenable to treatment with diuretics to correct the water metabolism and drugs which make the balancing organ less sensitive. It is rare before middle age.

Large quantities of aspirin taken by mouth will also produce a ringing in the ears. It is rare for large quantities to be necessary unless the treatment is specific as in rheumatoid arthritis or in rheumatic fever. When ringing in the ears begins it means that the aspirin level in the blood has reached a sufficiently high concentration to have an active effect in arthritis and rheumatic disease of the heart. Aspirin causes ringing in the ears because it affects the nerve for hearing, the eighth cranial nerve.

Ears, Wax in The external-ear canal is supplied with glands which secrete wax to keep the external ear well lubricated and moist. Ear wax is also a strong antiseptic and prevents infection in the ear canal. It is also water repellent and helps to stop the lining of the canal becoming wet and soggy. There is a tendency in childhood, and in certain individuals in later life, to secrete more wax than normal and the wax collects in dark brown lumps and may block the external auditory canal. When this happens the patient becomes aware that his hearing is muffled; a typical description is: 'I know I'm putting my feet on the pavement but I cannot hear them.'

You should never try to remove wax from your ears yourself, either by putting anything in the ears like hot oil drops or foreign instruments like hairclips, or wads of cotton wool – it is too easy to puncture the ear drum. You should go along to your general practitioner who can easily remove the wax by syringing the ears out with warm water.

Eczema Eczema is a chronic inflammatory condition of the skin which may start in infancy and involve the face and inner sides of the elbows, knees and wrists. It can be a cause of great distress not only to the affected baby but to the parents. The baby may be unable to stop herself from scratching during the night, quite often making the skin bleed, and it may be necessary to bind or glove the hands so that the baby cannot injure herself. The skin tends to be dry and crack easily. There is often a family history of eczema, asthma, allergies, migraine or travel sickness. All these conditions are thought to be related, and expressions of the same sensitivity in different ways in different individuals.

The outlook for infantile eczema is pretty good. More than half the children affected are free of eczema by the age of seven. The tendency for eczema to recur, however, usually remains throughout life, though it may take a different form in adulthood. It is usually seen as round, dry, red, scaly patches in the skin which come and go. Exacerbations of eczema can be caused by tonsillitis, an infection of any sort, a shock, stress, overwork, anxiety, a serious illness, an operation, a fractured limb, etc. and they nearly always take several months to settle down again.

A special form of eczema which is confined to the greasy areas of the skin is called seborrhoeic dermatitis and affects the scalp, the eyebrows, the folds round the nostrils, the ears and the front and back of the chest, and occasionally the groin and armpits.

There is no doubt that severe eczema requires special hospital treatment, but there are quite a lot of things that you can do for yourself in your own home.

1 You can, for instance, try to avoid contact with water as much as possible. Water, especially hard water, is a drying agent, and anything which dries an eczematous skin will make the condition worse. The first treatment we prescribed in hospital for a case of acute eczema was discontinuation of all washing and bathing.

2 Stop using soap of any kind. The cleaning action of almost every soap is achieved by a defatting process, and any agent which removes the surface layer of protective oils from an eczematous skin will irritate it.

3 If you have eczema of the hands, never wear rubber gloves for longer than five minutes, and never wear rubber gloves without a pair of cotton gloves underneath. If you do, your hands will sweat and in sweating they lose a great deal of moisture. When you take off the gloves and your skin dries out it will be more dehydrated than it was before, and the skin will crack very easily.

4 If you have to wear rubber gloves for household tasks, wear a pair of cotton gloves inside, and smother your hands in a mild hand cream or a special cream that your doctor has prescribed for you, so that the inside of the cotton gloves becomes soaked in cream. This way, when you wear rubber gloves, you are giving your hands treatment instead of doing them harm.

5 Ask your doctor to give you a special kind of moisturizing ointment which can be put in your bath. When this ointment is put in hot water it disperses into fine globules on the surface of the water, and coats your skin with a soothing emollient coating which will help to keep it moist and to prevent itching. It will also help prevent the drying action of the water.

6 Try not to wear any fabrics which are rough and prickly as this will irritate your skin and make you scratch; scratching injures the skin, making your eczema worse.

7 Try and avoid any situation where you may get overheated. When this happens the blood-vessels in the skin dilate and the skin becomes red and irritable, and your eczematous patches will get more itchy and inflamed.

8 Besides using the special cream that your doctor prescribes for you that contains powerful anti-inflammatory agents, you can use any bland emollient cream on your skin, as long as your doctor approves of it. Rub it in as often as you like. This helps to keep the skin moist, supple, cuts down itching and prevents dryness and roughness.

All of these things help to keep your eczema in a subdued state.

Eye, Chemicals in If the chemical is corrosive, like acid or bleach, hold the person or child, forcibly if necessary, with their head under a running tap and ask them to open their eyes. If they will not, try and get the help of someone who will open the eyes so that they can be washed out. If the chemical is not corrosive, wash out immediately with plain water and continue for some minutes. As soon as these manoeuvres are completed, take the person to hospital.

Eye, Foreign body in If you can see the foreign body, hold the upper and lower eyelids as wide apart as you can without causing too much discomfort (using the finger and thumb of your left hand) and remove the foreign body with the corner of a clean handkerchief. If the foreign body cannot be seen, try to dislodge it by pulling the upper lid over the eyelashes of the lower lid.

If this remedy does not work, try bending the upper lid backwards over a matchstick by pulling on the lashes of the upper lid. Sometimes this reveals the foreign body stuck to the upper eyelid or high up on the eyeball. In either of these cases, remove the foreign body with the corner of a clean handkerchief.

If this is unsuccessful, repeat the manoeuvre of exposing the upper eyelid, and wash out the eye with a solution made from one teaspoonful of salt and a pint of water. If the foreign body is still there you can do no more and the patient must be taken to the nearest hospital casualty department.

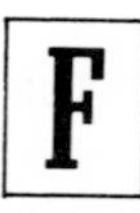

Fainting In Geordieland the term 'blackout' was used to describe loss of consciousness, regardless of cause. Blackouts therefore included fits, epileptic fits, concussion from a blow to the head, and strokes. The blackouts that will be discussed here are those which would come into the category of variations from normal, and so would include fainting from shock or fear, fainting during the early months of pregnancy, fainting from jumping up quickly from a kneeling or bending position, or fainting after a long soak in a very hot bath.

In all of these situations, the loss of consciousness or blackout is due to insufficient blood reaching the brain. When the brain is starved of blood it is starved of oxygen, and when brain cells are starved of oxygen they stop functioning and we lose consciousness.

The blood-supply to the brain may be reduced by mechanical or hormonal causes. Mechanical causes include those where the supply is cut off or is relatively diminished. The blood-supply is cut off when we crouch for a long time, because crouching kinks the blood-vessels in the legs, thereby trapping an enormous amount of blood in the lower part of the body and leaving only a small volume to serve the rest of the body. When we suddenly jump up, gravity pulls the blood down into the lower parts of the legs and also prevents the blood in the veins getting back up to the heart and thence to the brain, and so for a few seconds the brain is relatively starved of blood. That is why quite often we experience dizziness, if we don't actually faint.

Another mechanical reason why blood does not reach the brain in sufficient quantities is diversion to the skin. This happens when vessels become dilated over the whole surface of the skin. In this instance, more than half the body's blood is diverted to the skin, leaving half the normal volume to support the rest of the body. Dilation of skin vessels occurs whenever the skin is red, for instance when we lie in a hot bath, or when we take a lot of alcohol, or when we exercise and become very hot, and the blood-vessels open up to allow us to sweat and to cool down the body temperature. In any of these situations, jumping to your feet or trying to perform sudden physical movements can lead to a temporary depletion of the brain's blood-supply and you may experience dizziness or you may actually faint.

Fainting in pregnancy is due to a mixture of mechanical and hormonal causes. The mechanical cause is dilation of the blood-vessels which occurs in a pregnant woman to cope with the extra volume needed to supply her developing baby, her enlarging womb and the placenta. The blood therefore carries less oxygen than normal. The hormonal cause is progesterone which produces dilation of the blood-vessels of the skin, the pelvis and the womb. Both these factors lead to a relatively insufficient supply of blood to the brain. This can be aggravated by the moments of hypoglycaemia (low blood sugar) which occur in pregnancy due to the rapid utilization of the mother's sugar by the developing baby. The combination of hypoxia (low blood oxygen) and hypoglycaemia can cause a blackout.

Feet complaints Most feet complaints stem from lack of care of the feet and may start in childhood with badly fitting shoes and socks. You can wear fashionable shoes and still have trouble-free feet if you follow certain commonsense guidelines, because the key is to give your feet a bit of freedom.

1 Always choose your shoes with care, make sure they fit properly and don't hurt anywhere.

2 Try and change your shoes at least once a day; wear fairly sensible shoes for work, different shoes for driving the car, and again different shoes for evening, for dancing, walking, gardening, etc.

3 Wash your feet every day.

4 Change your socks or stockings at least once a day.

5 You should go barefoot as much as possible and encourage your children to do the same thing. Babies, of course, should never wear shoes.

6 Go to a chiropodist if you have serious foot troubles because over-the-counter remedies can be harmful if not used properly; even a corn plaster can give trouble if you have bad circulation.

7 Never wear anyone else's shoes, and don't hand down shoes from child to child – this will only encourage the development of corns and callosities.

(See also **Athlete's foot, Bunions, Warts.**)

Fever (Pyrexia) A fever is one of the commonest complaints that you are ever called upon to treat. Any fever over 101 °F. (38 °C.) should be taken very seriously and active methods used to try and bring the temperature down. It is your doctor's job to find out the cause of the fever, so consult him immediately.

It is important to lower the temperature because the body is made to function at 98.4 °F. (36.8 °C.) and will malfunction at a higher temperature. At very high temperatures brain cells cannot function properly and so the patient may become delirious and even pass into a coma.

First aid

Most temperatures can be lowered by the following methods:

1 Removing all clothing and bed covers.

2 Giving hypopyrexial drugs; aspirin is still the most potent drug we have for lowering temperatures and should be given in a soluble form, two or three tablets every four hours in adults, or according to the manufacturers' or your doctor's instructions.

3 Sponging the body all over with tepid water and not drying it, but allowing the water to evaporate off the skin. As it evaporates, it uses up heat from the skin, thereby cooling it, and the blood, and bringing the temperature down.

4 Directing a fan on to the naked body of the patient.

5 Keeping the patient's room cool and well ventilated.

First aid General procedures:

1 Keep the patient lying flat.

2 Keep the head and body level.

3 Raise the head if the face is flushed.

4 Raise the feet if the face is pale and the skin is cold and sweaty.

5 Turn the head to the side if the patient is vomiting.

6 In this order examine the patient for: bleeding, cessation of breathing, shock, poisoning, wounds and lacerations, burns, fractures.

7 Keep the patient warm with a blanket.

8 Send for a doctor or an ambulance.

9 Do not give spirits as stimulants or any drugs at all.

10 If the patient is conscious give hot coffee or tea.

11 Keep calm and do your best to keep the patient calm.

12 Keep onlookers at a distance.

13 Keep the patient as cheerful as possible until help arrives.

Flushes The commonest cause of a hot flush of the skin is the menopause. The severity of hot flushes can vary from those which cause very little inconvenience and are hardly noticed at all, to those which colour the patient's skin bright red, leave the patient soaked in sweat and are embarrassing and debilitating. They may occur up to twenty or thirty times a day and may also prevent the person from sleeping at night. If hot flushes are as severe as this, they require special treatment with menopausal remedies which may contain hormones, and therefore can only be obtained from your doctor. They can bring relief from hot flushes in a majority of patients.

There is a condition of the skin of the face which resembles acne called 'acne rosacea' commonest in women in their late twenties and thirties in which the skin periodically flushes. These flushes worsen the underlying skin condition. In the dermatology clinic we used to give these patients the following helpful hints:

1 Never expose your face to a direct source of heat such as a fire.

2 Try to avoid drinking hot drinks and eating any hot food.

3 Avoid highly spiced foods which may make you sweat such as curry.

4 Avoid extremes of hot and cold which cause the blood-vessels of the skin to dilate, or dilate in compensation after constriction.

5 Try not to go out in extremely cold weather as the skin tends to glow and flush when one comes indoors after being outside.

These tips will also help menopausal women who are having hot flushes. (See also **Menopause**.)

Food poisoning If you eat food that is contaminated with bacterial toxins you will have symptoms within an hour of swallowing the food – usually profound vomiting. If you eat food which is contaminated with bacteria, it will take longer for the symptoms to appear, probably several hours – and there will be vomiting and abdominal pain. If you eat food that contains only traces of bacteria, it may take up to twenty-four hours for the bacteria to multiply and cause symptoms which will probably be abdominal pain and diarrhoea, because the food has got further down the digestive tract. However, these situations may overlap, and food poisoning often causes diarrhoea and vomiting at the same time.

Depending on the virulence of the organism which is contaminating the food, the patient is in danger of becoming rapidly dehydrated due to the loss of fluid through vomiting and diarrhoea. There is the added danger of hyperpyrexia, and most importantly, danger from the toxins liberated by the infecting bacteria, which may affect other organs in the body from the intestine.

A case of mild food poisoning can be treated at home, and needs the same remedies as those given under **Diarrhoea** and **Vomiting**. A more severe case will need treatment with antibiotics from your doctor, and a very severe case will require treatment in hospital.

If a patient with food poisoning becomes very pale and his skin feels cold and clammy or if consciousness becomes abnormal in any way, call an ambulance and send the patient to hospital as he requires urgent treatment.

Fracture You can usually tell if a bone is fractured by the following simple test: ask the person to move the part where the bone is thought to be broken. If they can and do move the part, there is probably no broken bone. If they are unwilling or cannot move the part, then it is possible that a fracture has occurred.

Never try to move a suspected fractured bone yourself. The first step is to get help. The second step is to immobilize the injured part by splinting it. In extreme circumstances, this can be done by binding the fractured leg to the good leg, or the fractured finger to an adjacent good finger. Many common materials, however, make good splints; for instance, rolled newspaper. Do not move the patient until expert help arrives. If they are very pale and shivering, try to lower the head below the level of the rest of the body and cover them with a blanket. Do not give alcohol or stimulants, but a warm drink is in order.

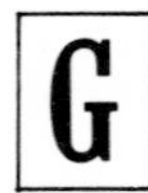

Gallstones If you're fair, fat, female and forty, and suffer from attacks of fatty indigestion, a pain under your right ribs which occasionally passes up to your right shoulder blade, then the chances are you are suffering from gallstones. Gallstones are collections of cholesterol, and are present in around a third of those who reach the age of seventy. Occasionally they cause inflammation of the gall bladder and give rise to the symptoms just described. Sometimes they may become impacted in the main bile duct, when they cause a very severe pain, gallstone colic, or biliary colic, which has the same characteristics as renal colic (see **Colic**). If the gallstone is not dislodged and the bile duct freed, then the escape of bile into the gut is blocked, and this will produce jaundice.

Chronic inflammation of the gall bladder causes attacks of flatulence, distension, especially after meals and especially after eating fatty foods, heartburn and right-sided pain. If there is a fever with these attacks, it means that the gall bladder has become infected and antibiotic treatment will be prescribed to bring the attack under control within twenty-four to forty-eight hours.

As there is no medicine which can completely dissolve a gallstone once it is formed, they can only be removed by surgery. Surgery for gallstones usually involves the complete removal of the gall bladder. This operation is called cholecystectomy.

Gastric ulcer see **Peptic ulcer.**

Gastritis Gastritis means acute inflammation of the lining of the stomach and the symptoms are very similar to those of a hangover, that is, loss of appetite, nausea, flatulence, acid indigestion, possibly heartburn, and possibly vomiting.

The treatment for any inflamed organ is to let the organ rest, so no food should be taken, but plenty of drinks; no active medication is necessary but a mild antacid from your chemist may help.

If the gastritis is part of a viral illness, e.g., flu, aspirin should be avoided as it may cause more irritation; paracetamol is the analgesic of choice. If it is accompanied by prolonged vomiting call your doctor. (See also **Diarrhoea**.)

Gingivitis Gingivitis is inflammation of the gum margins around the teeth. The commonest cause is plaque but it may be caused by bacterial infection. One of the most common and tenacious infections is a condition called Vincent's angina or trench mouth, which is contracted by drinking from an infected cup or glass. The bacteria become so deeply embedded in the pockets down the sides of the teeth that the only way to eradicate this infection is to perform a gingivectomy and to cut away the gum margin. The gums have marvellous powers of regeneration and by using soft wood sticks and gently massaging the gums between the teeth, they can be encouraged to grow up to their normal level.

Gingivitis may also be a side effect of certain drugs, for example, the hydantoins which are used in the treatment of epilepsy, and people who are suffering from lead poisoning often have a characteristic blue line around the gum margin which is diagnostic of their condition. The best way to prevent gingivitis is by attention to oral hygiene and proper brushing of the teeth (see pp. 79–81).

Glandular fever Glandular fever is characterized by swollen glands all over the body as the name suggests, a very sore throat which may be persistent and excruciating, a characteristic pinhead rash all over the body, and an enlarged spleen which you will not be able to feel but which your doctor will. Even the best physicians have been known to confuse this condition with a severely infected sore throat caused by the bacterium streptococcus, and allergy to penicillin, which is given to treat the former condition. It is only when neither get better that the diagnosis of glandular fever may become apparent.

Glandular fever is caused by a virus; its diagnosis is clinched by a special laboratory test done only in hospitals, and there is no specific treatment. The condition can be fairly debilitating. Many patients complain of mild depression, inability to concentrate, and general feeling of lethargy and lassitude for several months after the condition has cleared.

Glaucoma Glaucoma is a condition of the eye which is rare in people under thirty-five and increasingly common as age advances. There is nearly always a hereditary link and other members of the family may have had it.

The symptoms are fairly classical with pain starting in the eye and spreading over the head to give a severe headache. Vision may become misty and classically rainbow rings appear around distant objects. The eyeball is hard to the touch, though this may be difficult to detect by anyone except a practised physician. The eye may be pink and inflamed, though not always.

As glaucoma can damage eyesight if untreated, a doctor should be contacted as a matter of urgency.

Gonorrhoea see **Venereal disease.**

Gout Gout is caused by a hereditary abnormality of metabolizing proteins. It usually appears in men over the age of forty-five (though William Pitt had it at twenty-one) and is very rare in women.

The acute attacks usually start at night with excruciating pain in the big toe (large joints like the knee can be affected too); the joint is shiny, swollen and purplish red in colour and so agonizing to the touch that the patient will not even allow clothes to come in contact with it.

The attack can only be controlled with specific medicines, but the comfort of the patient can be helped by keeping him in bed with the affected foot slightly raised on a pillow and a special cradle placed over it to keep off the bedclothes. The patient should try to drink plenty of fluids – five or six pints a day – preferably water, but squash or weak tea will do.

With modern medicines pain should be relieved within twenty-four to forty-eight hours and the acute attack should have completely subsided in a week. If the gout is chronic then it may be necessary to take special medicines continuously and to adhere to a prescribed diet, not only to prevent recurrence of an attack, but to keep the weight on the low side.

Gum boil see **Abscess.**

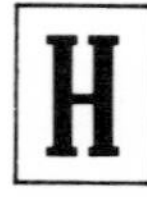

Halitosis Halitosis means unpleasant-smelling breath. The following conditions most commonly contribute to halitosis: being a mouth breather (as opposed to a nose breather); smoking; poor oral hygiene; infections of the gums, e.g. gingivitis, pyorrhoea; an empty stomach; not having taken drinks for some time, e.g. on waking in the morning; chronic alcoholism; chronic sinusitis; eating garlic, i.e. aromatic substances in the blood-stream are excreted by the lungs.

Even after excluding or correcting all of the above, halitosis may remain, in which case the condition can only be ameliorated by the use of antiseptic mouthwashes, sucking chlorophyll tablets, or as a last resort, minty sweets to mask the smell.

Halitosis should not be confused with the smell of acetone (pear drops) on the breath; the latter is a sign that diabetes is out of control.

Hangover To most people a hangover means a blinding headache, nausea, dizziness and thirst. The last symptom is the clue to what causes most of the horrors of a hangover – yes, thirst. Alcohol in fact 'dries out' your body. Your hangover is due, in part, to lack of water.

The explanation is that in getting rid of all the drinks you had, especially if they included 'fortified' wines like port, sherry and Madeira, your body uses up an awful lot of water and it draws on the water in your tissues.

It helps a little if you alternate water or fruit juice with your tipple and it is even better if you can swallow a pint of water before you go to sleep. But by far the best advice is everything in moderation. Avoid salty and sweet nibbles – they only contribute to the dehydration later. Take no more than two drinks an hour and drink fruit juice if you can. Fruit juice keeps you hydrated and gives you vitamin C which is also used when you metabolize alcohol.

Remedies for hangovers? – two fizzy vitamin C tablets, honey in warm water, two paracetamol and, yes, Fernet-Branca may help. Pet cures? – ice cream, watercress, and persimmon fruit. *Don't take any aspirin* (or any tablets containing aspirin, they only make the nausea worse and it may cause bleeding from the stomach lining if it is inflamed after taking alcohol: alcoholic gastritis).

Is there any truth in the belief that a hair of the dog that bit you can help? The answer is yes, partly, and the reason is interesting. The balancing organ in the inner ear (see p. 37) goes awry when there is a lot of alcohol in the blood but the body adjusts to that, given time. However, when all the alcohol has been cleared out of the blood the same disturbance hits the balancing organ a second time, hence the hangover. So by taking a little drink, and the emphasis is on *little*, you can slightly raise the blood alcohol level and give the balancing organ more time to get back to normal.

Hay fever Hay fever is caused by an allergy to pollen, and the symptoms of sneezing, red tearful eyes, blocked nose with profuse watery nasal discharge appear when the particular pollen is in season. Hay-fever sufferers are rarely allergic to only one pollen, the allergy usually involves several.

Symptoms can be relieved by antihistamine tablets but these may cause drowsiness which is dangerous if your profession necessitates your being constantly alert. Steroid drugs, particularly those given locally in spray form to the nose, may also be highly effective. No patent drops or sprays should be used without a doctor's instructions as they can damage the nasal lining. A recent treatment can help hay-fever sufferers by preventing the allergic response to pollen; it is only available from your doctor and is called sodium chromoglycate. By having a course of desensitizing injections during the six months prior to the expected appearance of your allergy, you stand a fifty-fifty chance of becoming desensitized to your particular pollen, but it has inherent dangers in that it may cause a serious allergic reaction.

If you are a hay-fever sufferer, you are asking for trouble if you go out into the countryside on a hot windy day during the season when your pollen is in the air. The best form of prevention is to avoid the causative agent.

Headache All of us suffer from headaches every so often, and frequently enough to recognize the various types of headache: the tension headache which feels like a tight band around the head; the migrainous headache which usually involves one side of the head and is accompanied by nausea and visual disturbances; the headache which occurs at ovulation or just prior to menstruation and is a dull ache at the back of the head; the headache which is centred over either or both eyebrows and is symptomatic of frontal sinusitis; the headache which accompanies viral infections like flu, which is the dull ache of toothache; the bursting, throbbing headache of a hangover, which is usually due to lack of fluids. All of these headaches cause discomfort, but are transient and self-limiting, and can be treated quite satisfactorily with fairly mild analgesics or specific remedies as in migraine.

The headaches which should be taken more seriously are those which: are unrelieved by analgesics; are continuous and unrelenting; start out of the blue when headaches have previously been rare; are of increasing frequency and severity; are accompanied by other symptoms such as loss of vision or pins and needles in the face or hands or feet or unsteadiness of gait, or vomiting. These sort of headaches require your doctor's attention and investigation. (See also **Migraine**.)

Head injury Anyone who suffers a head injury should be taken to hospital for an X-ray of the skull, whether they lose consciousness or not. Even if the doctor in the casualty department feels it is unnecessary to keep them in for observation, you should observe the person who has had a head injury yourself for at least twenty-four hours. You should be on the lookout for three things: a headache of increasing severity; the appearance of lumps or bumps on the scalp; a gradual loss of consciousness. If any of these things occur, call an ambulance immediately. Do not give drugs to any person who has had a head injury. (See also **Concussion**.)

Heartburn see **Dyspepsia.**

Heat stroke Under normal conditions the temperature of the body is regulated by a beautifully balanced mechanism which controls the amount of heat lost from the body. (Metabolic processes which are proceeding in the body all the time are producing heat and the main problem which confronts the body in maintaining homeothermic conditions is the loss, not the retention, of heat.)

The skin is the organ mainly in control of body temperature. It takes orders from the temperature control centre in the brain. When we are hot it does three things: it opens up its blood-vessels, allowing the blood in them to cool on contact with the air; it sweats, and the sweat takes heat from the body as it evaporates; it relaxes the muscles which make body hair stand on end to trap a layer of insulating air next to the skin when we are cold.

In heat stroke the skin is so badly burned by the ultra-violet radiation in sunlight, and the damage is so extensive, that it can no longer perform its function of controlling the body temperature. The body temperature soars and the temperature control centre in the brain is unable to correct it. In heat stroke, the temperature control centre has usually been damaged by excessive exposure to the sun. As it is situated on the base of the brain, that is the back of the neck, this part should always be covered by a hat or scarf when exposed to strong sun, especially in children. In theory, the body temperature could rise until death and the patient is in great danger from the moment consciousness is impaired by delirium or deepening coma. Heat stroke is therefore a medical emergency and a doctor should be contacted immediately or the patient taken straight to hospital whichever causes the least delay.

Hiatus hernia The symptoms of hiatus hernia, which are similar to those described under peptic ulceration, are caused by the reflux of the acid stomach content into the lower part of the oesophagus or gullet, but unlike the stomach, the lining of the oesophagus is susceptible to the corrosive action of the acidic gastric juices, resulting in inflammation and pain. Reflux can occur because the junction between the oesophagus and the stomach is imperfect and is worsened if intra-abdominal pressure is increased for any reason such as coughing, straining at stool, carrying heavy bags, or if the patient bends or lies down flat.

The treatment is as for duodenal ulcers and one additional measure which may help is to use three or four pillows at night; the upright position does not permit reflux of the stomach content into the oesophagus.

Hypothermia Hypothermia describes the condition where the temperature of the body *core* falls below normal. The body core is made up of all the vital organs in our body and includes the lungs, heart, brain, and nervous system.

It is newborn babies and the very old who are most in danger from the serious effects of hypothermia. New babies who are chilled are lethargic and unwilling to feed. The skin is very cold to touch and their body temperature is below normal. Their limbs, hands and feet may be pink and swollen. In old people the effect of hypothermia is similar with the same lethargy and apathy, and the lack of interest in food and any form of activity which can eventually lead to total immobility. If they are not re-warmed they may fall asleep and gradually lose consciousness and die.

Hypothermia was first recorded during the war. It was noted that shipwrecked sailors who survived after being picked up out of the water and taken to a host vessel – they even sat wrapped in blankets drinking hot cocoa – sometimes died a short while later. It was not understood why. It was only much later that we learned they had died from the effects of hypothermia.

Hypothermia must be treated carefully and slowly. The reasons why sailors during the war died was that their bodies were reheated too quickly. This meant that the outer layer of their body became warmer than the body core which remained at a low temperature. Crucially important blood was diverted to the outer warmer layer, leaving the essential organs deprived of blood and unable to function properly; death therefore ensued. We now know that re-warming must be a very slow process indeed. The best way of all to achieve it is to immerse the patient in a warm bath so that the body core can warm up at the same rate as the outer layers of the body. Warming a patient up too quickly can kill them.

I

Impetigo Impetigo is a disease of schoolchildren and, being infectious, can spread easily from one child to another in class. The surprising thing is that the bacterium which causes impetigo is an everyday inhabitant of the skin. It only causes impetigo when the surface of the skin is weakened by a scratch or knock, or when the numbers of bacteria on the skin multiply as they may in the damp conditions around the mouth and nose of children, especially in summer.

Impetigo forms easily recognizable bright yellow pustules which turn into scabs and then come off without leaving a scar.

The first line of treatment is with local antibiotic creams and possibly antibiotics by mouth prescribed by your doctor, but careful hygiene will help to clear the condition and prevent its spread.

Hygiene measures mean the face should be gently cleaned with the lather of an antiseptic soap and gently rinsed off. The application of an antiseptic lotion such as pHisoHex may also help. There should be scrupulous hygiene of the hands of the infected children and all those who touch them. Flannels, towels and nail brushes should all be thoroughly washed or rinsed in antiseptic after use.

Indigestion see **Dyspepsia.**

Influenza Influenza is caused by the influenza virus which can take many forms. Indeed in one year there can be half a dozen different forms of the same virus, which accounts for having more than one attack of influenza a year. The body builds up specific antibodies to the original virus which are useless in overcoming an infection by a variant of that virus. Flu injections are only partially effective because the antiserum which you are receiving can be effective against only a limited number of viruses.

The symptoms of influenza are well known – fever, headache, sore throat, cough, running nose, aches and pains all over the body, loss of appetite and a general feeling of lassitude.

While the temperature is high you should stay in bed and keep the room at a fairly constant temperature. Don't eat if you don't want to, but drink plenty of fluids. Take analgesics for your headaches and aches and pains in the form of two or three paracetamol every four hours. Suck any sort of sweet which will lubricate the throat; antiseptic throat pastilles are of limited use and local anaesthetic pastilles should not be used as they have a great propensity for causing allergies.

For an ordinary attack of flu there is no need to call your doctor as he can do no better than you can treating yourself in the manner described. If, however, you have any medical condition such as bronchitis or heart trouble where influenza might affect your general state, then you should always inform your doctor of an attack. If an attack of flu is not improving in two or three days or if your temperature remains raised, call your doctor.

Influenza virus usually enters the body through the lining of the throat and then circulates into various parts of the body. The same virus can give a variety of symptoms according to the part of the body which it affects most; so while it may produce the classical syndrome already described, it may also simply cause a high temperature, a headache and aches and pains in the muscles, particularly of the back and legs; or a sore throat and a honking, dry cough; or sneezing, nasal discharge and watering eyes. It may go down on to the chest and cause bronchitis, or it may concentrate in the stomach and lead to loss of appetite, nausea and even vomiting. If it concentrates in the bowel it will give rise to loss of appetite, abdominal pain and diarrhoea.

Ingrowing toenail see **Nails**.

Insomnia Insomnia is the inability to sleep. This may take the form of difficulty in getting off to sleep, waking in the middle of the night and not being able to go back to sleep, or waking early in the morning, wideawake, ready for the day and unable to go back to sleep. Not all of us need the same amount of sleep and you are only suffering from insomnia if you are getting less sleep than your body needs and you find yourself irritable, bad tempered, unreasonable and generally difficult to live with.

There is a special form of insomnia which occurs in pregnancy and may be one of the earliest signs of pregnancy, and is probably associated with the hormonal changes that occur as soon as the placenta is formed. Pregnancy has the effect of speeding up your metabolism and prevents the normal slowing-down process which occurs late at night.

The commonest causes of insomnia are worry, anxiety, overactivity (particularly just before going to bed), and intellectual activity (an example would be working flat out on a piece of work to meet a deadline and then going straight to bed – it is not surprising that the brain continues to work at full speed and you lie in the dark with your mind racing). Research has shown that the commonest feeling which prevents sleep is *resentment*; resentment against your partner, resentment that you are not getting a fair deal, resentment against your boss at work because he favours someone else, resentment against a neighbour because they have been unreasonable, etc. Reflecting resentfully on the events of the day will certainly stop you from sleeping.

Just as the inability to relax intellectually will stop you from sleeping so will the inability to relax physically. If you direct your attention to the state of your body when you are lying there unable to sleep, you very often find that it is tense, muscles are contracted, even your eyes and face may be screwed up.

There is no magic cure for insomnia, but here are a few of the remedies that have been found helpful:

1 Prepare for bed. Prepare your mind and your body. Have a bedtime routine which winds you down: making sure, for instance, that all the doors and windows are closed, making a pot of tea, collecting the newspapers and magazines that you might read in bed.

2 Prepare your bedroom. Make sure that it is well ventilated and neither too hot nor too cold. Make sure that you have a mattress in good condition and not a lumpy one.

3 Try to find some form of muscle-relaxing routine. You might even try yoga before you go to bed; some people find a short walk is good, lying in bed for fifteen minutes scanning the newspapers, or reading a chapter of a novel, or even watching television in bed, may produce the soporific effect you are looking for.

4 Make sure that all the squeaky doors are closed and all dripping taps are turned off.

5 Make sure that your nightclothes are not tight or constricting in any way.

6 A warm drink will help some people go to sleep, but it does not have anything to do with preventing night starvation, which is a myth. Don't eat a heavy meal just before going to bed; it can produce abdominal discomfort, possibly indigestion and may produce fitful sleep.

7 When you finally do turn the light off, go through a relaxation routine. Concentrate hard on each part of your body starting from your feet upwards and make sure that each part is relaxed. Then think about your breathing, try actively to slow down your breathing by taking slow, deep, regular breaths.

8 And a personal trick which I have found useful is to think of black velvet. It has the effect of emptying the mind and preventing thoughts from creeping in.

9 And here's one for a sleepless child. When I was a girl my mum used to tell me to 'try to think of the nicest thing that could possibly happen to me' – a new party dress or an exciting outing and to concentrate on that. I found this worked for me when I was a child and I went off to sleep untroubled, happy and contented. If it's not too naïve for you, try it.

10 Everyone can carry on with a few sleepless nights or a few short nights, but no one can carry on in the long term if they are not getting their quota of sleep. You must get sleep otherwise you will just not be able to lead a normal life and that is unfair on your family and your employer if you have a job. So seek help from your doctor and he will almost certainly help to re-establish your normal sleeping habits with the prescription of some sleeping tablets. You should try not to take these in the long term as you may get dependent on them, but just to see you over a bad patch and back to normal again.

Itching see **Pruritus.**

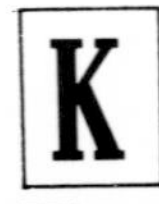

Kiss of life The kiss of life is the best way of giving artificial respiration to someone who has stopped breathing. You have only a few seconds to get air into the lungs so do not delay.

1 Lie the patient down on his or her back.

2 Open up the airways by supporting the back of the neck in your left hand while pressing down on the forehead with your right. If you have help, push the angle of the jaw forward from behind.

3 Take the deepest breath you can. Hold the patient's nostrils closed so that air cannot escape through the nasal passages and press your lips around his mouth (if it is a small child you will be able to get your mouth over the nose and mouth).

4 Exhale gently for as long as you can until his lungs begin to fill with air.

5 Repeat this half a dozen times.

6 If breathing does not start up continue to inflate the patient's lungs every four or five seconds.

7 Get the patient to hospital as soon as possible.

CARDIAC ARREST

If, besides not breathing, you notice that the skin around the patient's mouth is becoming blue, perform the following tests quickly:

1 Feel for a pulse. This is strongest and most obvious in the neck where the carotid artery runs behind the side of the Adam's apple.

2 Examine the pupils. If there is no pulse and the pupils are dilated, then the heart has stopped beating.

You can perform the following first-aid measure to try to restart the heart:

1 With your right hand, punch the chest fairly hard in the region of the lower end of the breast bone on the left side.

2 Repeat again within a few seconds if nothing happens.

3 If still nothing happens, kneel to the right of the patient. Place the palm of the right hand on the back of the left hand. With the 'heels' of both hands, pressing as firmly as you can (and sit up on your knees and put the whole weight of your body behind it), push down on the patient's chest at the lower left margin of the breast bone. Press down firmly, fairly sharply, and then release the hands.

4 Repeat this manoeuvre once every second until the patient's skin becomes pinker.

5 Check the carotid pulse to make sure the heart is beating.

If you have to perform cardiac massage and the kiss of life at the same time, inflate the lungs by mouth to mouth breathing once every six pressings with your hand.

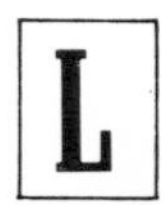

Laryngitis Laryngitis is inflammation of the voice box; the voice may become hoarse or it may be lost altogether. If it is part of a common cold or influenza, the treatment should be as for those conditions. If it lasts for more than a few days go and see your doctor for investigation of the cause.

Lice Lice can strictly speaking affect any part of the body but have a predilection for the hair of the head and the pubic region. Lice in the head (*pediculosis capitis*) is commonest among school children and one infected child can infect another when they put their heads close together in the classroom or playground. Contrary to popular belief, head lice prefer clean heads to dirty heads, and are just as happy in short hair as long hair. The lice lay their eggs (nits) at the root of the hair and make them secure with a cement-like substance which makes them difficult to remove with anything but a special comb. The eggs grow with the hair and take about six weeks to hatch out.

The most effective treatment is to apply a lotion which will kill both adult lice and the eggs and then only one application is needed. If you can allow the lotion to dry on the hair, thereby becoming more concentrated, the cure will be nearer a hundred per cent. The lotion is available from chemists. NB All members of the family should be treated at the same time and all members of the family should be checked for reinfestation in three or six weeks.

Pubic lice (*pediculosis pubis*) is usually contracted by venereal contact. The treatment is the same as for head lice. All consorts should be treated and checked for reinfestation.

Loss of weight Excluding slimming regimens, some of the commonest causes of loss of weight are:

1 Acute illnesses, especially if there is fever, vomiting or diarrhoea.
2 Digestive disorders that are aggravated by taking food, e.g. gastric ulcer.
3 Difficulty in swallowing from any cause.
4 Diabetes mellitus.
5 An over-active thyroid.
6 Pulmonary tuberculosis (now very rare).
7 Any cancer or cancer-like illness, for example, leukaemia.
8 Anorexia nervosa and other nervous disorders.

The treatment is the treatment of the underlying conditions. Your doctor should be consulted to arrange for investigation of the cause.

Lumbago see **Back pain.**

Lump in the breast see pp. 92–3.

Lump in the throat (*globus hystericus*) The sensation that there is a lump in the throat is most common amongst over-anxious, fussy, middle-aged women, and is largely imagined (hence the *hystericus*). The true organic cause is hardly ever revealed even by the most exhaustive investigation.

The sensation that there is a hair in the throat, which may be sufficient for the patient to resort to using all sorts of strange objects to remove the hair, thereby scratching the back of the throat to the point of bleeding, is also of the same nervous and imaginative origin.

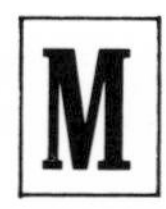

Menière's disease see **Ears, Ringing in.**

Meningitis Meningitis is usually due to a viral or bacterial infection and, whatever the cause, it requires hospitalization. Here are a few simple pointers to look for if you suspect that someone in your house is suffering from meningitis and which, if absent, may prove a source of reassurance. If you are in any doubt, however, call your doctor immediately.

1 The cry of a young baby with meningitis is often high-pitched and screaming, quite unlike the baby's normal cry.

2 Adults always complain of severe headache.

3 A child or adult is sensitive to light and will turn the face away from any sort of light, even daylight, and will ask you to draw the curtains and switch off lights. This sensitivity to light is called photophobia.

4 Meningitis means inflammation of the meninges which are the fine paper-like coverings of the brain and nerves. When they become inflamed it is painful if they are stretched and the muscles of the back and head may go into spasm to prevent it. Another simple test for meningitis, which can complicate the viral infection of poliomyelitis, was used during the polio scares of the forties and fifties: ask the person to put their chin on their chest. If they can manage this without too much discomfort ask them to bring their forehead down to their knee. If this causes severe pain, or is prevented by muscle spasm, meningitis can be clearly suspected.

5 The temperature of course is always high and the patient may have a convulsion and may lose consciousness. If either of these things occurs, call your doctor immediately, or get the patient into hospital as quickly as you can.

Menopause The menopause is the cessation of menstruation, and may occur at any age over forty, but is very rare under the age of thirty-five and is most common during the late forties and early fifties. It can happen in several ways: the periods may still occur every month but become scantier; the loss of blood may remain about the same but the periods become less frequent, though not haphazard, say every four weeks, then every six weeks, then every eight weeks, etc.; a combination of the first two patterns. *Any other form of irregular vaginal bleeding is not a normal part of the menopause and you should consult your doctor.*

The menopause is caused by the ovaries becoming inactive and failing to secrete normal amounts of female hormones. This may cause women no trouble whatsoever, or may give rise to the most disabling symptoms, the commonest of which are: hot flushes; emotional changes, e.g. tearfulness, anxiety, insecurity, profound depression; loss of intellectual function, e.g inability to concentrate, inability to deal with problems, failure to make decisions; loss of libido (sex drive); changes in the genital tract, e.g. drying, irritation, itching of the vagina and external genital organs which leads to dyspareunia or pain on sexual intercourse.

Women may experience none, any or all of the above symptoms. If they are serious enough to prevent you coping normally with life, then you should consult your doctor for help. There are now available special treatments to help you cope with the hormonal shortage that your body is experiencing, and special menopause clinics that you can go to for help and advice with, of course, your own general practitioner's approval.

If the symptoms are very disabling ask to be referred to a gynaecologist for specialist advice and do not be palmed off with the statement that the menopause is a perfectly normal event and you should be able to cope with it without any treatment. (See also **Flushes**.)

Menstruation Menstruation starts with the menarche (at any age after about eleven) and ends with the menopause.

Well before the age of eleven all girls should have a full explanation of menstruation and the implications of it. It should also be pointed out that the first period is rarely in the form of red blood but is more likely to be brownish or black. A young girl should also be told about dysmenorrhoea (painful periods), that this occurs in about fifty per cent of women and is serious in only a very small percentage. It usually starts the day before menstruation begins and clears with the establishment of the menstrual flow. They should be discouraged from thinking that dysmenorrhoea is a disabling condition or needs any more treatment than simple analgesics. Two paracetamol every four hours while the pain lasts should be enough. Discourage retirement to bed with a hot-water bottle; it is much better to be active. (See also **Colic**.)

Frequent heavy periods (menorrhagia) usually occurs in mature women and there is nearly always an underlying gynaecological cause which can be treated. Your doctor's assistance should therefore be sought.

Lack of periods (amenorrhoea) may be primary or secondary. Primary amenorrhoea means that the onset of menstruation – i.e. the menarche – is delayed. In most cases there is no underlying cause and menstruation becomes established during the teenage years. Occasionally primary amenorrhoea is due to a hormonal imbalance which needs investigation by an endocrinologist, so you should consult your doctor who will refer you to the specialist.

Secondary amenorrhoea is lack of menstruation after having had regular menstrual periods. The commonest cause is pregnancy and this should always be ruled out with a pregnancy test. Secondary amenorrhoea often turns out to be delayed menstruation. Delay can be caused by a profound change in your life such as anxiety, overwork, stress, worry, jet travel, fear of pregnancy, a serious illness, an accident, a shock, etc. Amenorrhoea which lasts more than six months should be fully investigated by a gynaecologist or an endocrinologist.

Migraine Migraine is the unilateral headache whose pain is stabbing in character and which is often preceded by visual disturbances, such as: partial loss of vision, blurring of the outline of lighted objects, and spots before the eyes. The headache may be accompanied by abdominal symptoms which range from nausea, profuse vomiting to abdominal pain. Occasionally the abdominal components may be more dramatic than the headache when the mistaken diagnosis of appendicitis may be made.

Migraine sufferers are typically obsessive, meticulous, highly intelligent, highly sensitive people and stress very often plays a part in the causation of the headaches. However, all migraine sufferers will report that they have periods when they appear to be 'sensitive' to the headaches and have them frequently, without any exacerbating factor that they can put their finger on. On the other hand, they can go for long stretches when they appear to be 'resistant' to the headaches, and conditions and circumstances which previously brought on incapacitating attacks leave them quite free of pain.

Most migraine sufferers also describe that the headache usually comes on when the stress is over, when they let up, when they relax, when the hard work has been done and the effort made. It is as though some mechanism in the body keeps them going until it doesn't matter and, when they are free of the stress, the headache comes on.

Headaches can last anything from a few hours to several days and during this time the patient can be prostrate and will claim that the only remedy is to lie absolutely still in a darkened room and sleep if possible. Eating is unthinkable, and drinking may be difficult. It is nearly always impossible to keep down analgesics or specific migraine remedies. If, however, one can take a tablet of the ergotamine variety with the onset of visual symptoms, one may be able to abort an attack. A long-time migraine sufferer may learn to abort an attack until after the pressure lets up by exerting 'mind over matter'.

The Migraine Trust (45 Great Ormond Street, London WC1) has done a great deal of research into migraine. Whilst we know a great deal about it we still do not know the specific cause, though we do know that the visual symptoms are caused by the constriction of the blood-vessels of the head, and the bursting headache is caused by the dilation of the blood-vessels which occurs after the initial phase of constriction. Sometimes the constriction of the blood-vessels may be so great and so generalized throughout the brain that the common symptoms of numbness and tingling, running of the nose and the eye and the corner of the mouth on the side of the head which is affected by the headache is superseded by paralysis of the side of the face, and even of the whole side of the body.

Motion sickness Motion sickness, migraine, eczema, asthma and allergies are all thought to be connected, and form a hereditary pattern of reaction to stress, be it physical, chemical or emotional, which shows itself in different forms in different individuals.

Motion sickness is a hypersensitivity to disturbance of our balancing organ. This balancing organ is found in the inner ear and sends information to the brain of the exact position of all parts of our body and minute changes in their position. The eyes, of course, can give visual information about the same thing. Motion sickness occurs when the eyes send the brain one message and the balancing organ sends the brain another. Confusion arises because the messages from the eyes are instantaneous whereas the messages from the balancing organ, which are transmitted by the movement of fluid, are necessarily slower. Thus the message from the balancing organ arrives at the brain several seconds after the appropriate message from the eyes, by which time the eyes are sending a different message. The result of these conflicting messages is a feeling of sickness.

The logical treatments would be to:

1 Cut down the information that is passed to the brain by the eyes, i.e. close the eyes.

2 Diminish the sensitivity of the balancing organs to movement, and this is how travel sickness pills work.

3 Minimize the changes in position of the body by lying down.

If you suffer motion sickness take a pill *before* travelling according to the instructions on the pack. You may still feel nauseated but you probably won't vomit.

Mumps Mumps is a virus condition which involves certain glands of the body. In children these glands are the salivary glands which swell up in the neck and cheeks and are so painful that swallowing and eating may be prevented. In adults, however, the virus causes inflammation of the ovaries and the testicles. This is extremely uncomfortable and fairly serious because fertility is interfered with in a small percentage of patients. A case of mumps in an adult always requires a visit from the doctor, and special fertility tests after the infection has subsided if your doctor thinks it is necessary.

Simple analgesics such as paracetamol will ease the discomfort and the sufferer should be given soft minced foods through an invalid feeding cup with a spout to make swallowing easier. Acidic foods, e.g. citrus fruits, should be avoided, they cause salivation which is very painful if the salivary glands are inflamed as they are in mumps.

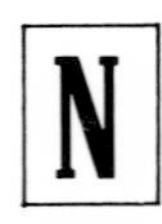

Nails Most trainee doctors are told that a close inspection of the nails can reveal a good deal about the health of their owner, and indeed there are certain medical conditions which can be diagnosed from the appearance of the nail, for example: spoon-shaped nails (koilonychia) are characteristic of iron-deficiency anaemia; pitting of the surface of the nail so that they resemble the surface of a thimble is characteristic of psoriasis; thickening and yellowing of the nails which are lifted up from the nail-bed is also characteristic of psoriasis, but may also be found in fungal infections of the nail; a white line across a nail or a ridge which gradually grows out marks a serious illness or a severe shock; enlarged rounded over-curved nails, 'clubbing', is symptomatic of chest diseases; a blue line in the nail is characteristic of lead poisoning; small red flecks in the nails are 'splinter haemorrhages' and are characteristic of certain types of heart disease and a group of diseases affecting the arteries.

All these signs can be seen in the toenails as well as in the fingernails but there is one condition which is specific to the toenails. This is an ingrowing nail. One can try to prevent a toenail from becoming ingrown by making certain that the nail is cut straight and not down at the side. If a toenail grows in persistently and is causing pain, it may need to be removed. You should consult your doctor about having this simple, minor operation done.

The nails, like the hair, are dead so there is nothing you can apply to them to make them more healthy. You may strengthen them by applying hardeners but their health depends on your health and eating a well-balanced diet.

Nausea see **Gastritis, Motion Sickness, Peptic Ulcer, Vomiting**, and *Miriam Stoppard's Book of Babycare* for nausea of pregnancy.

Nettle rash (Hives, Urticaria) Nettle rash can be diagnosed by anyone because it is the only rash which lasts ten minutes and disappears completely. The spots in the skin are exactly the same as those which occur after you are stung by a nettle – that is raised, round, oval spots about the size of a pea surrounded by a flare in the skin which are excruciatingly itchy.

The causes of chronic recurrent nettle rash are legion. The underlying mechanism is usually one of allergy. It is necessary to investigate your case in a hospital clinic and find out to what you are allergic. Having found it, the only cure is to avoid it. Symptomatic treatment, however, may be quite successful. On the skin you can use a cooling lotion such as calamine lotion; antihistamines by mouth will also help. In children a common cause of nettle rash is flea bites. The child becomes allergic to the fleas and nettle rash appears in parts of the body distant from the flea bite. The treatment in these cases is to get rid of the fleas – and usually the cat or dog as well.

Nits see **Lice.**

Nosebleeds Nosebleeds usually occur from the lining of the nose just inside the nostril where the blood-vessels are very close to the skin. They can therefore easily become damaged by friction, by a knock, or by increasing the pressure in the nose, e.g. blowing the nose.

Nosebleeds occur most commonly in childhood and middle age. In middle age they may be symptomatic of increased blood-pressure and should always be investigated by your doctor.

The first treatment of a nosebleed is as follows:

1 Never put the head backwards; it only allows the blood to trickle down the back of the throat and into the stomach where it is an irritant and will cause vomiting.

2 Always put the head forward over a sink or receptacle if possible.

3 Apply gentle pressure on either side of the nostrils.

4 Cooling with ice on either side of the nostril may speed up the cessation of bleeding.

Numbness (and pins and needles) Numbness and pins and needles are usually from two causes: the nipping or obstruction of an artery; or the nipping of a nerve. An example of the former would be the numbness and tingling we feel after having our legs crossed for a time, when the artery behind the knees is compressed. An example of the second would be sciatica when a slipped disc may press on the sciatic nerve root.

A mixture of both would be the 'metacarpal tunnel syndrome'; this occurs most often in middle-aged women and is due to a band of tissue across the front of the wrist tightening, compressing the blood-vessels and nerves, giving rise to numbness, tingling and pain in the fingers. It is always most severe at night. It can be relieved by a minor operation.

Very occasionally the sudden onset of numbness or tingling in a particular part of the body like one hand, one foot, or a side of the face can be symptomatic of a special group of nervous diseases which need investigation by a neurologist and you should consult your doctor about these symptoms if they occur out of the blue.

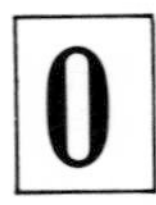

Obesity see p. 45.

Overdose see **Poisoning**.

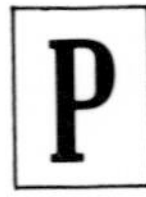

Pain As a general rule, any severe pain lasting longer than half an hour warrants advice from your doctor and the same can be said of an excruciating pain for any length of time.

IN THE ABDOMEN This could be appendicitis, diarrhoea, diverticulitis, dysmenorrhoea, duodenal ulcer or gastric ulcer.

IN THE BACK see **Back pain.**

IN THE BACK OF THE LEG Sudden pain in the calf which is worse when you try to draw up the foot, accompanied by swelling of the leg and ankle, and tenderness when pressure is applied, may be due to a deep vein thrombosis. You should rest the leg immediately by going to bed if possible, and call your doctor who will visit you to examine the leg, and give you the appropriate treatment.

Superficial pain in the leg accompanied by redness of the skin may be due to a superficial thrombophlebitis, that is a small thrombosis in one of the superficial veins of the leg. This is nearly always accompanied by infection which tethers the clot to the wall of the vein so that it cannot escape. Again you should rest and immobilize the leg, and call your doctor who will give you specific treatment.

IN THE CHEST This may be cardiac in origin, but it is just as likely to be due to indigestion, wind, gallstones, viral infection of the muscles of the chest wall, spontaneous pneumothorax, pleurisy, duodenal ulcer, gastric ulcer or one of several other causes which have nothing to do with the chest itself.

IN THE EAR see **Earache.**

IN THE KNEE If you have pain in the knee and there is nothing apparently wrong with the joint, consult your doctor because disease of the hip may cause pain which is referred to the knee.

ON BREATHING This is symptomatic of bronchitis, tracheitis, pleurisy and fractured ribs.

ON COUGHING This is characteristic of pleurisy, tracheitis and fractured ribs – indeed severe coughing can fracture a rib!

ON PASSING A STOOL The commonest cause is an anal fissure which is a tear in the lining of the back passage, usually caused by passing a large stool or a hard stool. The pain of an anal fissure may be exquisitely severe and many patients believe that they are suffering from cancer. Patients with anal fissures have been known to take their lives in this belief. This condition can be completely cured by injection or minor surgery, so consult your doctor.

ON PASSING URINE see **Cystitis.**

For those pains not severe or prolonged enough to call the doctor do the following:

1. Lie down.
2. Take analgesics (aspirin, paracetamol) as directed on the pack.
3. Undertake no exertion.
4. Avoid excitement or anxiety.
5. Apply local heat.

Palpitations Palpitations is racing of the heart, and the speeding up of the heartbeat can be felt by the person experiencing palpitations.

Palpitations has several causes: a shock, nervousness or anxiety, indigestion or gallstones, an over-active thyroid, high blood-pressure, angina or any kind of heart disease. While there may very well be no detectable reason, the condition should always be investigated by a doctor. However, there is one manoeuvre you can try for yourself. Take in a very deep breath and hold it for as long as you can. This has the action of slowing down the heartbeat and may stop your attack of palpitations.

Parkinsonism (Parkinson's disease) This is a condition more common in men than in women, and is due to the effect of hardening of the arteries on certain parts of the brain. The face has a mask-like appearance and there may be a coarse tremor of the hands when they are at rest, with the fingers going in one direction and the thumb in another, the so-called 'pill-rolling effect'. There is a tendency to stoop and walk with short quick steps. There is a tendency to salivation and for the mouth to stay open. The handwriting of a person suffering from Parkinson's disease is characteristically small and gets smaller as the disease progresses.

New treatments can relieve muscle spasm and tremor. Certain measures that you can take for yourself involve exercising as much as possible (beneficial exercises learnt from a physiotherapist can be continued at home), and carrying things such as a newspaper or a rolled umbrella to help diminish the tremor.

Peptic ulcer This is a general term which includes duodenal ulcers and gastric ulcers.

DUODENAL ULCERS Duodenal ulcers are caused by an excessive secretion of acid in the stomach. The stomach is impervious to the amount of acid it contains because it has a special lining which protects it. The duodenum, however, does not and if there is an excess of acid the lining of the duodenum may become inflamed, swollen, damaged and eventually ulcerated. If the ulcer is not treated properly it may become enlarged, erode a blood-vessel and cause a haemorrhage, erode into the pancreas which lies behind the duodenum, causing severe pain in the back, and distort the architecture of the duodenum so that the outlet from the stomach is narrowed down to a very small hole, thereby permitting the sufferer to take only very small amounts of food if he wishes to avoid vomiting.

Doctors do know that certain factors make a duodenal ulcer worse, and exacerbating factors include: going for long periods without food; eating a rich fatty diet; taking large amounts of alcohol frequently; smoking any cigarettes at all; being overworked, worried, under stress and going without sleep.

Those steps which help a duodenal ulcer were discussed under the heading of

Dyspepsia; in addition, the following points have been proven beyond doubt in several very well-conducted research studies.

1 If you are a smoker, the quickest way to heal your duodenal ulcer is to give up smoking altogether. This has been proven beyond a shadow of doubt.

2 The second best thing that any person suffering from a duodenal ulcer can do is to rest. Whilst most people who must lead an active life cannot do this, there is no doubt that absolute and complete rest will heal a duodenal ulcer in six weeks, given that the person isn't smoking.

Most physicians and surgeons agree that the above two factors are the most important ones in keeping a duodenal ulcer under control and curing an acute attack. One small tip worth repeating is to keep a glass of milk and a biscuit by your bedside; if you should have an attack of pain in the middle of the night it will be relieved by sipping the milk and chewing the biscuit.

In the last two years a new drug, cimetidine, has been discovered which can prevent the excessive secretion of acid in the stomach of duodenal ulcer sufferers and that drug can completely change the life of many people who suffer from this ailment. It is of course only available from your doctor.

GASTRIC ULCERS Gastric ulcers can be distinguished from the duodenal type because the pain comes on *after* taking food whereas the pain from a duodenal ulcer is *relieved* by taking food. As part of your treatment your doctor will probably recommend a special diet and provide you with a diet sheet for guidance.

Phobias A phobia is a profound, though irrational, fear of certain situations. Even though a person is aware that they are behaving stupidly, they are unable to control the fear. The fear can be related to an earlier, possibly distressing event which has been forgotten, and experiencing this fear may be accompanied by physical symptoms such as sweating and even vomiting. Most patients suffering phobias recognize their fears as excessive and unreasonable but are unable to quell them and quite understandably they are prepared to go to great lengths to avoid their phobic situation, even to confining themselves completely to their own home if they suffer from fear of open spaces (agoraphobia). Among the commonest phobias are: acrophobia (fear of heights), ailurophobia (fear of cats), anthophobia (fear of flowers), anthropophobia (fear of people), aquaphobia (fear of water), arachnophobia (fear of spiders), brontophobia (fear of thunder), claustrophobia (fear of closed spaces), cynophobia (fear of dogs), equinophobia (fear of horses), microphobia (fear of germs), murophobia (fear of mice), mysophobia (fear of dirt), ophidiophobia (fear of snakes), pyrophobia (fear of fire), thanatophobia (fear of death). About eight out of every thousand people suffer from a phobia to a degree. Disabling phobias occur in one or two per thousand people.

There are now many ways of successfully treating phobias which involve group therapy and psychoanalysis. The first fear you have to overcome is the one to visit your doctor to ask for help. But please do so because you can be helped.

Photophobia see **Meningitis**.

Piles Piles are varicose veins of the rectum. The primary cause is an inadequacy of the valves in the veins of the rectum which allows blood to run backwards and pool. However, piles only cause trouble if other factors are added to the primary defect: pregnancy, where the pressure of the developing baby makes pooling of the blood in the rectal veins worse; chronic cough where the increase in abdominal pressure forces the blood back into the rectal veins; chronic constipation where straining of the stool causes an increase in the abdominal pressure and promotes pooling of the blood in the rectal vein. (See also **Varicose veins**.)

When piles become large enough to prolapse outside of the anus, they can cause quite a lot of trouble in the form of itching, soreness and pain. If one of them becomes nipped off, pain can be extremely severe. Usually the piles can be pushed back into the rectum with a greased finger and will remain in place. If, however, piles are prolapsed for any length of time they require active treatment either with injections, which will make them shrivel, or surgery, when they will be stripped out.

Pins and needles see **Numbness.**

Poisoning If the person who has taken the poison can tell you what it is and it is a non-corrosive poison such as a medicine, try and make them sick by tickling the back of the throat, or making them drink a concentrated salt solution (two heaped tablespoons to a half pint of water). If the poison is corrosive, for example, disinfectant, your efforts should be directed towards diluting it by giving large quantities of water or milk to drink.

If the patient is unconscious but still breathing, lay him on his side with the lower arm placed behind the body and the lower leg slightly bent upwards at the knee. Put something underneath the neck so that the head is held on its side and is tilted slightly downwards from the level of the rest of the body so that the tongue cannot be swallowed and choking is prevented.

If the patient is unconscious but still breathing, lay them on his side with the lower airway to make sure it is open and then proceed with mouth-to-mouth resuscitation (see **Kiss of Life**). If the patient is comatose or is sinking into a coma, and there is any evidence that sleeping tablets, anti-depressants, tranquillizers, or aspirin (one of the most dangerous) have been taken, especially if with alcohol, call an ambulance and get the patient to hospital at once.

Pre-menstrual tension To the well-known symptoms of pre-menstrual tension like breast tenderness, a feeling of distension in the abdomen, lower abdominal pain, tearfulness, irritability, extreme hunger, nausea, vomiting and weight gain can be added worsening of such diseases as epilepsy, acne, asthma and eye disease, rheumatic pains, skin rashes, hay fever and nettle rash. All are part and parcel of the syndrome which women suffer in the days preceding menstruation and in the early days of menstruation. Not only is the above list of symptoms fairly generalized throughout the fertile female population, but recent work by Dr Katharina Dalton has shown that good loving mothers may become baby batterers during the pre-menstrual period, that illnesses and accidents are not just more common in the mother suffering from pre-menstrual tension, but also in her children, husband and immediate household, that women tend to drink more (or the effects of alcohol are greater) in the pre-menstrual period and that the incidence of crime and psychiatric illness is greater.

Like the menopause, this is a female complaint which tends to be treated rather lightly by doctors. But if your pre-menstrual syndrome is disabling to yourself and your family, you should seek medical help.

Dr Dalton found that the most efficacious treatment was progesterone, and the best results are obtained if an inplant is placed painlessly underneath the skin. If you nannot obtain treatment from your own doctor, diplomatically but firmly ask for referral to an endocrinologist or a gynaecologist.

Pruritus (Itching) Itching of the skin nearly always occurs as part of another condition (for example, jaundice, eczema, nettle rash, insect bites or fleas) and treatment of the itching should be part and parcel of the treatment of the primary condition. The application of a cooling lotion such as calamine lotion will always help suppress itching, and antihistamine tablets from the doctor may help too.

There are two specific instances of itching which are worthy of note because they are the symptoms of fairly serious but treatable conditions. The first is itching in the genital region after passing urine which may be symptomatic of diabetes mellitus, and is due to the high concentration of sugar in the urine. The second is itching in the genital region accompanied by an unpleasant vaginal discharge; this is nearly always due to a vaginal infection. If you suddenly begin to experience itching of the vaginal region, consult your doctor. Genital itching can have psychological origins, as can any itch. Do not apply local anaesthetic creams because they can cause an allergy.

Pyelonephritis see **Cystitis**.

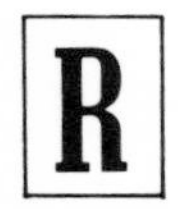

Rashes Rashes are patches of redness in the skin which may be anything from a pinhead to the size of a dinner plate, which can be flat or lumpy, which may disappear on pressure or not, which may last minutes or years and in their general form, pattern and distribution may act as diagnostic flags to an experienced doctor. There are so many of them that to describe each one is beyond the scope of this book, but their treatment, with the exception of those rashes which are the manifestation of skin disease only, extends beyond local application and involves treatment of the underlying condition by your doctor.

As far as local applications are concerned, here are some general rules:

1 For cooling, use calamine lotion or any lotion which dries out.

2 For lubrication, use an oil-based ointment, e.g. vaseline.

3 For dry cracked skin, use a cream that will hold moisture in the skin, e.g. baby cream.

4 If the skin is weeping, keep it wet, bathe it in normal saline solution (one teaspoonful of salt to one pint of water) and apply wet lint dressings soaked in the solution.

5 If the skin is scabbed, do not remove the scabs but use dry dressings with an antiseptic talcum powder underneath.

6 If the skin is broken in a child or is in a 'dirty' area (for example, the hands), use an antiseptic cream, e.g. Savlon, applied three or four times a day.

Raynaud's disease (Dead fingers) This condition is due to a hypersensitivity to cold. When the hands are exposed to severe cold they first go white (dead fingers) then blue, then become bright red and very painful. The treatment is to keep the hands covered and warm. Youngsters who experience this effect when they go swimming should be excused swimming lessons.

Red eye see **Conjunctivitis** and **Glaucoma**.

Ringing in the ears see **Ears, Ringing in.**

Ringworm Ringworm is caused by a fungus infection and is commonest amongst schoolchildren. It usually affects the scalp but it can affect also the skin. In the skin the fungus infection starts as a red, itchy, scaly patch, which gradually extends. The centre heals, leaving a red scaly ring in the skin – hence the name. When the scalp is involved, circular patches of baldness appear as the fungus attacks and kills the hair growing in the follicle. Ringworm may also affect the groin, the beard and the feet.

The diagnosis is fairly straightforward if there are several cases about. If not, it can be confirmed by shining ultraviolet light on the skin or scalp when the patches will fluoresce green. It is the ringworm fungus which fluoresces green when exposed to ultraviolet light.

The treatment for ringworm is Whitfield's ointment (obtainable from your doctor) applied two or three times a day in a thin smear to the affected area, and meticulous hygiene of the clothing, flannels and towels that are used by the patient.

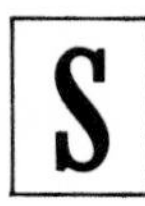

Scabies Scabies is a skin infection caused by a mite which burrows a centimetre or slightly more under the skin and lays its eggs at the end of the burrow. It has a predilection for the spaces between the fingers, round the wrists, the ankles and between the toes, but it may affect almost any part of the body if left untreated for a long time. The presence of the mite is very irritating and patients invariably complain of intense itching. Diagnosis is clinched by finding burrows which show as fine greyish lines, usually in the finger clefts, ending in small black spots. If a black spot is removed by gentle probing with a fine needle and examined under a microscope, it turns out to be the easily recognized adult mite.

The mite is highly infectious and may be picked up by venereal contact. Treatment involves painting the whole of the body with an application available on prescription. All members of the family must be treated.

Sciatica see **Back pain.**

Shingles Shingles is caused by a virus, herpes zoster. The virus homes in on and causes inflammation of nerves. The shingles virus is a close relative of the chickenpox virus and the rash is similar with small vesicles which eventually open, weep and then scab over. In shingles the rash is confined to the distribution of the nerve which is affected, so in a classical case when a spinal nerve is involved, the rash will girdle the body on the side affected. The rash is usually preceded by a burning pain along the part of the nerve affected and a few days later clusters of pearly blisters appear on a base of inflamed skin. After scabbing the rash may take two to three weeks to clear completely, but the nerve pain often persists for much longer.

Treatment is non-specific. One must keep the blistered skin dry with talcum powder or calamine, and relieve the nerve pain with analgesics. If the rash becomes infected, then one must apply an antibiotic ointment, available only from your doctor.

Shingles is particularly serious when it affects the nerve that supplies the eyeball as the blisters may cause ulcers of the conjunctiva. Ophthalmic herpes, as it is called, should have specialist treatment in hospital. In older patients it may leave a debilitating facial neuralgia which is very difficult to treat.

Shock Shock, in medical terms, is not the same thing as the lay description of someone who is shaken up, nervous, tearful and jittery. Shock to a doctor means a state of cardiac and circulatory collapse which endangers life. Shock is always a medical emergency. The patient is pale, the skin is cold and clammy, and there may be a bluish tinge around the mouth. Sweating can be profuse and, if not unconscious, the patient feels faint and giddy and states that vision is blurred. Breathing is rapid and shallow. If untreated, shock can lead rapidly to death. The causes of shock are always very serious, such as severe bleeding, either internally or externally, widespread burns, coronary thrombosis, severe injuries, a burst appendix, a perforated ulcer or a stroke. Send for help immediately. Staunch external bleeding by pressure, reassure the patient and keep them quiet and as comfortable as possible. Cover them with a blanket and keep the room fairly warm. Do not give them hot drinks or apply hot-water bottles. They quite often complain of profound thirst, in which case you should let them sip a cold water drink.

Sinusitis The commonest presenting symptoms of sinusitis are headache and a pussy discharge from the nose. There are six sinuses in the skull bones, three pairs arranged symmetrically: above the eyebrows, beneath the cheekbone, and on either side of the bridge of the nose. These sinuses are air cavities lined with mucous membranes. As they are enclosed spaces with only small exits, it is difficult to eradicate a bacterial infection from them and sinusitis is very often chronic. Even if it becomes quiescent, it can be triggered off again by any minor infection of the nose or throat.

Chronic sinusitis may result in a collection of pus within the sinuses which will show up if they are X-rayed. Treatment with drainage may be necessary, as well as prolonged courses of antibiotics, to which the infecting bacterium is sensitive.

Skin ulcer The commonest ulcers of the skin are varicose ulcers. These ulcers occur at the inner side of the ankle bone and are due to varicose veins. The ulcer is often preceded by a rough itchy patch of eczema which when scratched easily breaks down and then is difficult to heal and may spread to involve an area of skin four or five inches in diameter. Because the nutrition of the skin is so poor in this area, the ulcers take an extremely long time to heal and the outlook is poor as long as the varicose veins are present.

Most patients with varicose ulcers can be referred to the local dermatology clinic at which a whole morning or a whole day may be set aside for treatment of varicose ulcers. Routine hospital treatment is as follows, and there is no reason why a variant of it should not be followed at home.

1 The patient lies for half or three-quarters of an hour with the legs resting at an angle of 45° above the body. This drains all the fluid out of the legs.

2 The ulcer is then dressed with an appropriate antiseptic or antibiotic lubricant tulle, covered with dry gauze and then bound fairly tightly with a crepe bandage and possibly an elastic bandage on top. This dressing can be left intact for a week or more if the ulcer is not infected.

3 If the ulcer is infected, then it is carefully bathed with an antiseptic solution when the old dressing is taken off and, when the specific infecting organism is known, the appropriate antibiotic can be used on the ulcer to get rid of the infection.

The second most common ulcer of the skin is called a rodent ulcer and is commonly found on the faces of old people. It is a very, very slow growing ulcer and starts with a small shiny bump which gradually enlarges to form a ring with pearly edges and a clear inner circle. These small ulcers respond excellently to special X-ray treatment.

Slipped disc see **Back pain.**

Sore throat Sore throats may be caused by viruses or bacteria. Viral sore throats are more common and there is no specific treatment for them. Antiseptic throat lozenges should be avoided as they may disturb the normal bacterial harmony of the mouth and throat and they cannot cure virus infections anyway. Gargles are no longer generally recommended because it is thought they may spread the infection instead of curing it. The simplest remedy is to suck any sweet which causes salivation to keep the throat lubricated and to take mild analgesics if the soreness precludes swallowing. A liquid diet taken through a wide straw or an invalid's cup will help mealtimes to be more comfortable.

The commonest bacterium to cause sore throats is the streptococcus and the streptococcal throat has a classical strawberry-red appearance and may affect the tonsils. A streptococcal sore throat is amenable to penicillin treatment which if given will clear the throat of the infection in about three days, but a full course of five to seven days should be taken to avoid penicillin resistance in that strain of the streptococcus.

Sprains Sprains are usually caused by torn or bruised ligaments around an unstable joint such as the ankle or the knee. They are accompanied by pain, swelling (due to the accumulation of fluid), and limitation of movement.

The treatment for sprain first and foremost involves removing weight completely from the damaged part and rest. If the part is not completely rested, any other form of treatment will be largely ineffective. If the part is completely rested it can be back to normal within as short a time as three days. If it is not rested it may take six to eight weeks to return to normal.

Besides rest, the sprained part should be firmly bandaged with a cold-water compress, or some lint soaked in magnesium sulphate solution which will help to reduce the swelling and then firmly bound with a crepe or elastic bandage. Mild analgesics can be taken for the pain.

Stings see **Bites and stings.**

Stools Alteration in the appearance of stools may be a symptom of some internal disorder.

BLACK STOOLS see pp. 146–7.

BLOOD IN THE STOOL see pp. 146–7.

FLOATING, FATTY STOOLS Often seen as part of malabsorption syndrome, coeliac disease or cystic fibrosis.

PALE OR CLAY-COLOURED STOOLS Occur when there is blockage of the bile duct by a gallstone, and are usually accompanied by jaundice, the cause of which must be thoroughly investigated in hospital.

PENCIL, PIPE-LIKE STOOLS Due to a stricture in the rectum and you should always draw this to your doctor's attention.

SLIME IN THE STOOLS May be a symptom of inflammation of the bowel and you should always alert your doctor to this occurrence.

Stroke A stroke is nearly always due to a block in, or a haemorrhage from, one of the blood-vessels which are in the brain which has hardened or thickened. Before a complete block occurs there may be warning symptoms and mild attacks with transient confusion, spells of dizziness, difficulty in speaking clearly, a weakness or numbness and tingling in one part of the body, say a hand or a foot, slight dimming of vision which may last for several days. A severe attack with headache, confusion, vomiting, loss of vision, unintelligible speech and coma with paralysis of the whole of one side of the body or the upper or lower half of the body, means that there has been a vascular catastrophe in the brain.

If the patient is unconscious, leave them on the floor and put a pillow under the head. Remove false dentures, and turn the head on the side with the face pointing towards the floor so that vomit will not be inhaled. Whether the patient is conscious or unconscious, call your doctor urgently.

Though recovery is rarely one hundred per cent, with modern methods of treatment, such as that devised and advocated by Sir Ludwig Guttman at Stoke Manderville Hospital, based on mobilizing the patient as soon as possible, the outlook is very good. Improvements depend on many auxiliary nursing services, such as physiotherapy to get the patient moving and walking again, speech therapy to help them with speech difficulties, and above all, cheerfulness and confidence in the immediate family and encouragement for the patient to be persistent and determined so that his confidence and independence are restored.

Stye A stye is a pustule in the hair follicle of an eyelash. It often occurs in a person with an underlying blepharitis (chronic redness and inflammation of the margin of the eyelid) or with seborrhoeic dermatitis, and is generally interpreted as a sign of being run down. As the swelling arises and before the pustule forms, the stye can be very itchy but rubbing it only encourages its progression and may even spread the infection.

Do not touch or interfere with the stye and do not try to treat yourself. Seek a good antiseptic cream which is suitable for use in the eyes from your doctor.

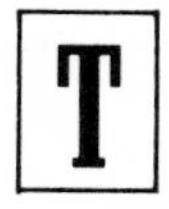

Tapeworm see **Worms.**

Thrombophlebitis see **Pain.**

Thrush Thrush is a fungus infection caused by a variety of yeast called candida, or monilia. Medical synonyms for thrush are candidasis and moniliasis.

Candida is a normal inhabitant of the whole of the gastro-intestinal tract and under normal conditions its growth is held in check by competition with the other bacteria in its environment. If the environment is changed, however, and the numbers of its competitors are reduced, as they are when long-term antibiotics are given by mouth, candida may overgrow and cause a thrush infection.

Thrush can give rise to symptoms in three main areas:

ANUS An itchy rash surrounding the anus spreads to involve the genital regions. The rash consists of small red lumps in the skin which may become pustular and the edge of the rash often has a wavy, scaly appearance as the yeast spreads out to infect more distant parts of the skin. The diagnosis is confirmed by taking scrapings from the edge of the rash and examining them under a microscope, when the yeast can be seen. This infection of the anal and genital skin is due to an overgrowth of candida in the gut and therefore the skin rash cannot be adequately treated unless the overgrowth in the gut is contained. It is therefore necessary to take a specific anti-candidal drug, Nystatin, by mouth, at the same time as treating of the skin, to completely clear the infection.

MOUTH Thrush of the mouth occurs most commonly in newborn babies. They catch thrush as they are born if their mother has an infection of the vagina. In a baby's mouth thrush is very difficult to distinguish from milk curd, but one does so by trying to remove the white patch. With milk curd it is easy, with thrush infection it is difficult and if one can remove it the lining of the mouth is left raw and bleeding where the yeast has been. The treatment for oral thrush is Nystatin solution which can be painted on the lining of the mouth with a cotton bud, and also Nystatin by mouth to clear any infection which has descended further into the bowel.

VAGINA Candida also naturally inhabits the vagina and if the biological population in the vagina is altered, then candida may overgrow and cause a thrush infection there. When the surface of the vagina is examined, it is red and inflamed and there may be small white specks which are clumps of growing yeast cells. There is nearly always vaginal discharge which is creamy yellow in colour, thick, and has an unpleasant odour. It causes itching of the genital skin outside of the vagina. Treatment for vaginal thrush is Nystatin cream or Nystatin pessaries.

Tongue complaints SORE TONGUE Nearly always caused by taking food which is too hot, but smoking, be it cigarette, pipe or cigar, if overdone, can lead to a painful tongue. A rough tooth or a plate, continually rubbing the tongue, can also lead to a sore patch which may eventually develop into an ulcer, in which case seek help from your dentist.

FURRED TONGUE Hardly ever a symptom of disease. The uppermost layer of the cells of the tongue is constantly and rapidly being shed. The action of eating and drinking removes the dead cells without trace. If for some reason such as an illness or an operation we do not eat for several hours, then the cells collect on the surface of the tongue and give it that yellowish-brown furry look. Contrary to popular belief, it is not a sign of indigestion or being run down.

BLACK FURRY TONGUE Due to a fungus infection which can be treated with gentian-violet paint.

SMOOTH TONGUE Without any of the papillae which make it rough, this is nearly always a symptom of pernicious anaemia (see **Anaemia**).

ULCERS OF THE TONGUE Can be APHTHOUS which arise spontaneously and are often related to a period of stress or overwork. They take ten to fourteen days to go through their whole cycle, are excruciatingly painful and unresponsive to virtually any form of treatment. They occasionally can reach an enormous size, say an inch in diameter, and really look rather frightening, but they heal very quickly. Most other ulcers of the tongue are caused by mechanical injury such as a sharp tooth, or a wire from a plate, or from the hot smoke of a pipe which is held constantly in one position in the mouth. Treatment of these ulcers of course is to remove the mechanical irritant. An ulcer which is caused by chronic irritation or heat, as from an old-fashioned clay pipe, can after twenty to twenty-four years go on to malignant change, so one should correct one's bad habits early and let the ulcers heal.

Tonsillitis The tonsils are two small glands situated at the back of the throat which have an active function only in childhood. They are part of the body's defence system and by trapping unwanted viruses and bacteria at the level of the throat, they prevent infection from penetrating further into the body. In performing this defence action, they quite often swell and may become infected. When they do so the upper glands of the neck may swell along with them and become tender to the touch. Tonsillitis is invariably accompanied by a sore throat and possibly by difficulty in swallowing which may be severe enough to prevent normal eating. The patient may have to revert to a liquid diet taken through a straw or invalid feeding cup.

The commonest form of tonsillitis is viral with a cough and nasal discharge. There is no specific treatment other than simple analgesics.

Streptococci are the second most common cause of tonsillitis when the throat appears cherry red and the tonsils may be greatly swollen with collections of yellow pus on the surface. This condition fortunately is amenable to treatment with penicillin which should be taken for a minimum of five to seven days. In young children tonsillitis may lead to a middle-ear infection or to bronchitis and so should always be taken seriously. Chronic recurrent tonsillitis which involves the ears or the chest, or is complicated by tonsillar abscesses is grounds for the removal of the tonsils, tonsillectomy. When this operation is performed, the adenoids are usually removed at the same time – 'T's and A's' (see **Adenoids**).

Toothache Toothache is nearly always due to tooth decay and may be preceded by sensitivity to hot and cold and sweetness, which means that the outer layer of enamel is damaged. You should consult a dentist as soon as you can. Meanwhile mild analgesics will help relieve pain, and a hot-water bottle will soothe. Painting the tooth with oil of cloves should be used only once or twice as too frequent use may result in damage to the gum margins.

Tracheitis Tracheitis is inflammation of the trachea with pain under the breastbone on breathing in or coughing. It is nearly always accompanied by bronchitis (see **Bronchitis**).

Travel sickness see **Motion sickness.**

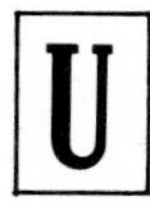

Ulcers: Duodenal see **Peptic ulcer; Gastric** see **Peptic ulcer; Skin** see **Skin ulcer; Tongue** see **Tongue ulcer.**

Urine There are many misunderstandings about the appearance and smell of urine.

Urine is light or dark in colour according to how much fluid you are drinking. If you are drinking a lot of fluid it will be pale, lemon-coloured and if you are not or you are in a very hot climate where you sweat a great deal, the urine will be a dark orange colour. Urine which is dark in colour is often described as being 'strong'. There is nothing wrong with 'strong' urine. Strong urine is entirely normal and is simply dependent on the amount of fluid available to be secreted as urine. If there is only a small amount of fluid available then the waste products which are excreted in the urine are concentrated, but healthy kidneys are perfectly able to cope with the situation, in fact they are especially designed to do so.

When the urine looks 'strong', it is said to smell 'strong'. It is bound to, because there is a higher concentration of waste products in it than when it is dilute. But this is perfectly normal too and there is nothing wrong with strong-smelling urine. When there is an infection present in the urine, it has quite a different smell and is easily detectable from strong, normal urine.

Urine may be very dark brown in colour due to a chemical called urobilinogen, and accompanies jaundice, or a condition in which the red blood cells are being rapidly destroyed, called haemolytic anaemia. The first is fairly common, the second is fairly rare but you must tell your doctor in any event. Blood at any time in the urine, be it bright red or dark red, is abnormal and must be reported immediately to your doctor. It should be remembered that certain dyes contained in food come out in the urine, for instance, the dark red dye of beetroot. Urine can take on the strange smell of things that one eats; synthetic penicillin, ampicillin, for instance, is concentrated in the urine and the smell is a most distinctive one of burnt rubber.

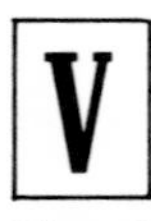

Vaccination see pp. 78–9.

Vaginal discharge see **Discharge, Vaginal.**

Varicose veins Varicose veins occur most commonly in the legs, but have already been described in the rectum under **Piles**; they may also occur rather infrequently at the lower end of the oesophagus, and usually secondary to cirrhosis of the liver.

Varicose veins in the legs are elongated, tortuous veins with irregularly distended walls and incompetent valves. In normal veins there are valves which allow the blood only to flow upwards and prevent it from dropping backwards. Varicose veins form after a major vein has been blocked by a thrombosis and branches open up to provide alternative routes for blood flow. One of the consequences of the thrombosis is that the valve in the thrombotic vein becomes damaged. Blood therefore soaks back and pools in the superficial veins which show on the legs as irregular dark-blue coloured compressible lumps.

While the symptoms of varicose veins like aching in the legs can be relieved by wearing elastic stockings, or by binding the legs with elastic bandages, the underlying fault can only be rectified by surgery. Surgical operation involves stripping out of the incompetent deep veins so that there can be no seepage back into the superficial varicosities. Any varicosities which may remain after surgery can be shrivelled up by painless injections. You can reduce the strain on your veins by making sure that you are not overweight, by always sitting instead of standing, by treating a cough and constipation promptly (both cause pressure downwards into the leg veins), and by keeping the foot of your bed slightly raised so that the fluid is always draining away from your ankles. When you are sitting always try to keep your feet resting on a stool.

Venereal diseases Venereal diseases are contracted during sexual intercourse. The two main diseases are syphilis and gonorrhoea, but scabies, pubic lice, herpes and other viral conditions may be contracted by sexual contact, as may some fungal diseases. Both infections are increasing in incidence. More seriously, the bacteria which cause syphilis and gonorrhoea are becoming resistant to standard methods of treatment.

If you suspect that you have venereal disease, contact the local citizens' advice bureau for the address of the nearest hospital which runs a special clinic. Patients may go directly to such a clinic without seeing their general practitioner and total confidentiality is maintained.

With syphilis, the first sign of the disease is a single painless ulcer which appears three to four weeks after you have had intercourse with an infected person. The ulcer may be on the penis or the entrance to the vagina, on the mouth, the nipple, the anus, or fingers.

With gonorrhoea, the first symptoms appear three to ten days after infection has taken place. There is severe pain on passing urine, and a discharge of thick yellow pus from the vagina or penis. If untreated the discharge may dwindle away and then reappear.

It is important to have both of these diseases treated rigorously and promptly because they are both associated with very severe complications as the disease progresses. Gonorrhoea may lead to sterility in a woman and strictures of the urethra in a man, which may need regular dilation with a metal dilator. Over a period of years, untreated syphilis will eventually involve the brain, rendering the sufferer insane. An untreated woman can pass syphilis on to her baby while she is carrying it and it will almost certainly suffer from severe physical malformation.

Both syphilis and gonorrhoea used to respond very successfully to penicillin. Both bacteria are now resistant to standard forms of penicillin and the search for new drugs is constantly going on.

Other venereal diseases include trichomonas vaginalis and thrush which can be treated simply and successfully (see **Thrush**). Part of the treatment of venereal disease should be the encouragement to take a responsible attitude to sex.

Verrucae see **Warts.**

Vomiting Vomiting is most often a symptom of gastric irritation – see **Diarrhoea, Dyspepsia, Food Poisoning, Gastritis** and **Peptic ulcer.**

Reflex vomiting occurs because the vomiting centre in the brain is stimulated and can occur with the following conditions: liver disorders; kidney disorders; appendicitis; gall bladder disease; pancreatic disease; migraine; pregnancy; after a general anaesthetic; urinary tract infections, particularly pyelonephritis; feverish illnesses such as measles and whooping cough; head injury; meningitis. In children with a raised temperature it may be due to any cause, but particularly with ear infections and tonsillitis.

Treatment is bedrest and nothing to eat or drink by mouth. As the vomiting ceases, sips of water may be taken and then milk diluted with water and then fruit juice diluted with water. If plain water induces further vomiting, a good tip is to try adding a teaspoon of salt to a pint so that it matches the body's own fluid and to continue sipping this solution until the tendency to vomit is over. If vomiting is relentless the patient must be taken to hospital so that fluid can be replaced by intravenous feeding.

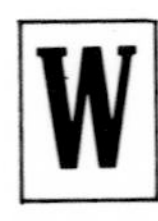

Warts Warts are tiny tumours in the skin caused by viruses. As has already been stated, the medical profession does not have a successful cure for virus infections and so warts can only be treated by scooping them out (curettage), by burning them out with fuming nitric acid, by freezing them to death with solid carbon dioxide, or by softening them and then scooping them out through the application of special corn plasters followed by curettage.

Warts occur most commonly on the hands and on the feet. Because of pressure from walking the warts on the soles of the feet (verrucae) tend to bury themselves into the skin instead of protruding from the skin as they do on the hands.

Verrucae are most common in children and are usually picked up in the swimming baths. They must be treated very carefully because if over-treated they may result in a scar and the scar can be more painful than any verruca and may last for the rest of the patient's life. So a verruca should be treated slowly and carefully.

Very occasionally warts form in the genital regions. These are very difficult to treat because they are moist, fragile and tend to spread quickly. They may take years to eradicate and must be treated by a specialist in a dermatology clinic.

Warts, of course, are self-limiting, that is why patent wart cures and 'magic' wart cures work. Most warts will disappear in about two years. This is because it takes two years for the body to build up antibodies to the virus. Once there are sufficient antibodies, the virus is killed off and the wart withers. When I was running a dermatology clinic, people came to see me who had had warts for eighteen months. I always tried charming them away, and in sixty per cent of cases I succeeded, not because of any charm that I had but because the body was on the point of developing its own treatment for the warts.

Senile warts appear on the face and the back of the hands in old people and are due to chronic exposure to sunlight. They usually require no treatment.

Water brash Water brash is the regurgitation of acid from the stomach into the mouth, normally after a heavy meal or rich food. The treatment is the same as for dyspepsia (see **Dyspepsia**).

Wax in the ears see **Ears, Wax in.**

Whitlow A whitlow is a small abscess down the side of the nail fold and hardly ever occurs unless the skin is very soggy, i.e. washerwoman's hands, or the skin is constantly being picked and torn as a nervous habit, and in addition to these two things, the standard of hygiene is very low.

The whitlow is very painful indeed and can completely prevent the use of the infected finger. Only rarely does the pus escape of its own accord. A serious whitlow must be treated in a hospital out-patients' department by lancing, scraping out the cavity of the infection and treating with antiseptic or antibiotic dressings.

Worms Worms are most commonly seen in the stools of children. In the United Kingdom the most common type of worms are threadworms, which may be quite numerous in the stool and look like short pieces of slow-moving thread and be anything up to half an inch long. One of the symptoms is itching around the anus, particularly at night because the adult worm comes out of the anus to lay its eggs on the surrounding skin.

Tapeworms, though not as common as they were, still infect children. They have flat paperlike segments which can be seen in the stool. The whole worm could be several feet long, but usually only single segments are passed. If the worm is long it can absorb large amounts of nutrients from the food and therefore the patient will suffer considerable loss of weight.

Human beings are the secondary host to tapeworms, the primary host being pigs. Humans contract the worms by eating pork which has not been cooked well enough to kill off the tapeworm cyst which is embedded in the meat of the animal.

If you spot either of these worms, or any worm, in the stool of your child, do not try patent medicines but take your child along to the doctor where you can be given specific radical treatment that will clear the stools of worms.

Wounds see **Bleeding.**

Index

Note: Page numbers of figures and tables are in *italic* type.